JUICING IN THE FAST LANE

THE ULTIMATE ROADMAP FOR JUICE BEGINNERS, DETOX, AND WEIGHT LOSS

B. L. GRUBBS

CONTENTS

INTRODUCTION

"Eat plenty of fruits and vegetables," your doctor says, "and make sure to exercise and get enough sleep!" Boy, if there ever was a more simple health recommendation that was harder to apply in real life, it would be this one! We now live in a time where the average person doesn't even get to shop for their food properly and think about their food choices, let alone eat enough foods that are being recommended. Seriously, commuting alone makes your workday a 12-hour journey, where you're lucky if you garner the patience not to pick up some cheeseburgers, and instead choose to munch on fried steak and some french fries.

You're not alone in your struggle to keep up a healthy lifestyle amid checking off to-dos. Plus, let's face it, eating fruits and vegetables can be so burdensome.

Even if you like them, there's always the issue of finding quality products and discovering the sweet spot when it comes to amounts purchased in order to avoid throwing away stale veggies that you never even got a chance to unpack. I've been there. Getting a health scare, and then taking the time after work to finally go to the grocery store and get some good quality food. The abundance of food there is mesmerizing, and within minutes, you see yourself as one of those buff, fit people lecturing others about how you used to struggle with healthy eating, unaware of how easy it was to change. Or, is it?

Some 30 minutes to an hour later, you're standing at the cash register with a "Pinterest-perfect" cart. There are all colors of the rainbow in veggies and fruits, and you've also discovered some nice supplements to further enrich your diet. You're packing your food at the parking lot, all empowered and just waiting to see your pounds shed and your energy spike. The first thing you discover after coming home is just how much energy it takes to cook all those foods. Boy, it doesn't seem like you've accounted for the expiration dates, and now it seems like you need to eat two weeks' worth of food in a single week. Nothing major, you can cook side dishes and freeze them, right? That's easy. You can even catch up on your favorite Netflix shows while doing that. Except for the fact that you have so many other chores and errands. There's a home to tidy up, kids to take care of, and you also need to get ready for tomorrow's presentation at work.

Fast forward two weeks ahead, and your fridge is empty... Again. You've thrown out almost half of your produce, and the dishes you cooked, while appetizing, aren't quite it. You're ordering takeout again. At times, it might seem as if changing your lifestyle is impossible. No matter how hard you try, getting out of your comfort zone and establishing new routines is difficult. I agree. Most of our health problems come from an irregular lifestyle and an imbalanced way of eating, sleeping, and moving. Diet appears to be the sore spot for anyone wishing to make a change. Whether you simply dislike fruit and vegetables, or you don't have the time to cook, you need a solution.

That solution could easily be a juicer. Why? In case you didn't know, juicing is a great way to eat tons of fruits and vegetables without actually having to eat them. Get a quality juicer, and you can squeeze delicious essences from pounds of fruits that will deeply replenish your body within minutes. Knowing just how beneficial juicing can be for overall health, and having improved personal health myself, I decided to publish Juicing in The Fast Lane. As the title suggests, this book is intended for anyone in need of positive nutrition changes, whose lives figuratively unfold 'in the fast lane.' Racing against the clock can rid you of the time needed for quality self-care, and a powerful juicer can help bridge the gap between what your body needs and what your itinerary allows.

In this book, you'll learn about the basics of juicing as a supplement to a healthy diet. First and foremost, you'll learn how juicers operate and how they're designed to extract the nutritious delight from almost any fruit or veggie. Then, you'll learn how to choose the juicer that's right for you. Not all juicers are the same, and as you're about to learn, the choice of your best machine depends on how much juice you'll make each day and which foods you prefer.

After learning the basics of what juicers are and how to use them, you'll also learn what foods are best recommended for juicing. We'll start with fruits, where you'll learn which common fruits benefit your health the most. You'll learn the same regarding the best vegetables for juicing. Despite the popularity of green juices and smoothies, people are still only vaguely aware of how much vegetable juice is beneficial for their health. Moreover, you'll learn about just how many veggies can be eaten raw that you didn't think about before. Lastly, you'll learn about delicious herbs that you can add to your juice to enhance its flavor and boost nutrition.

Altogether, the recommendations given in this book will empower you to use your juice for its best-intended purposes. You need to know how to juice correctly. Incorrect juicing has caused many people to dismiss it as a fad. Misconceptions about taking too much sugar with juice and drinking too many nutrients that your body can't process have led many people to give up on juicing overall. Not anymore! This manual will show you how to juice while keeping your daily calories at the lower end of the spectrum, and how to avoid taking too much sugar with your juice. More importantly, you'll learn where to find those rare, yet extremely beneficial nutrients that protect your body from chronic and life-threatening illnesses.

Lastly, you'll learn how to juice for specific purposes. In this book, you'll find easy recipes to juice for weight loss, detox, and healing from specific conditions and illnesses. You'll learn how juicing can benefit weight loss despite the misconception that it causes weight gain. You'll learn how to make low-carb and low-sugar juices that will support your digestive health and metabolism, enabling you to ditch processed sugar and forget about unhealthy snacks. Your body needs a decent cleanse as well. After years of unhealthy eating, your body's natural mechanisms that filter and expel toxins from itself may have slowed down. Such is the case with the liver and kidneys, which can begin to operate less efficiently under the burdens of too much blood sugar, high cholesterol, and hormonal imbalance. Juicing for detox can help you cleanse and reset your body, further supporting your organs in doing what they're meant to do all along– support your body's healthy functioning. Finally, you'll learn amazing juice recipes to recover from common ailments. Colds, allergies, aches, and pains trouble many people across the globe. While you should use the medical treatments recommended by your doctor, juicing can help reduce the symptoms and allow you to enjoy a better living quality while your treatments take effect.

So, what's there to wait for? Hurry up, and begin learning about all of the amazing ways to juice!

1

GETTING TO GRIPS WITH JUICING

D o you want to be in great shape and enjoy vigorous health without having to munch on vegetables? You're not alone! People all over the world are looking for a simple, hustle-free way to stay healthy and fit. So, why is it so hard? First, there are many people, like yourself, who don't enjoy eating healthy foods. We now know that many recipes that make healthy foods delicious also destroy their nutrients, so you're technically not getting all of the vitamins and minerals promised by the nutrition chart. Cook more consciously, and you end up spending a ton of time boiling and steaming veggies that taste bland. You might be conscious enough to know that this is the right way to cook, but you're not enjoying your meal. Soon enough, you're back to good-old plates of pasta and fried meals, with regret in your heart and cushions around your waist. Altogether, shopping, cooking, and prep time that goes into healthy recipes is just too much. You need a boost in your nutrition that's quick, simple, and tasty.

This is where juicing kicks in! This is a simple daily ritual that can help you achieve a nice-looking body, and quell those pesky sugar cravings by replacing snacking habits that are hard to shake with a quick dose of healthy sugars and a bomb of micronutrients. These nutrients, as you might guess, boost your immune system, help balance out your hormones, recover damaged health, and make you feel better overall. In this chapter, you'll learn exactly what juicing is, and how you can do it starting today.

THE JUICING BASICS

Why are so many people obsessed with juicing? To go back to basics, health nutrition is all about eating/drinking the foods that bring in maximum healthy nutrients into your body with minimum nega-tive effects that come from the build-up of fats, carbs, and sugars. It is a gentle balance, and arguably one that's becoming super difficult to attain. Now, how does one eat to get the most nutrients that build up their body and provide energy without going overboard with calories and sugars? As you have likely learned on your journey, the secret to that is eating lean, nutrient-dense foods and keeping your daily calories either the same as what you burn to maintain weight, or somewhat less if you wish to lose weight. The math is easy enough on paper, but really, who is to know how much you're eating when you saute or pan-fry vegetables, or cut random fruits into a salad? You find yourself lost, and you have no idea what you're doing since it's virtually impossible to keep up the nutrient logistics in real life. Juicing is a simple, healthy method to take lean nutrients in their purest form so that your body can break them down and use them more efficiently.

To understand why this is the case, you should first learn more about how your body absorbs nutrients. After you eat or drink, the foods get broken down into nutrients in your stomach. They are then distributed across your entire body and used to build and maintain cells, tissues, organs, hormones, neurotransmitters, and everything else that keeps your body functioning. When you don't have enough nutrients, you start to lack essential ingredients that create the substances needed for your body to work properly. This is when you start to see numerous symptoms, from tiredness to a weakened immune system. Your metabolism also slows down, and your body begins to operate with reduced capacity. When this happens for a long time, the effects of malnourishment can start to snowball into chronic illnesses, many of which take years to recover from, even with the best efforts.

Conversely, a healthy supply of nutrients gives your cells the substances that they need to regenerate. Circle back to how you're used to cooking and eating, and you'll realize that you're likely not getting enough essential nutrients, and you might even be eating too many fatty and starchy foods that further harm your health. Transforming your lifestyle has to start somewhere, and a simple switch from drinking sugary beverages to drinking only healthy, satiating juices might be the spark that ignites an entire chain reaction of healing from the inside out.

For many people who've struggled with health and metabolism, getting a juicer has had a transformative effect. This is because juicing allows you to start your day with a potent blend of nutrients from fruit and vegetable juice that gets absorbed quickly into your body. After all, your stomach doesn't have to do the extra work of digesting, and it can instead get straight into shooting nutrients into the cells that need to be healed and repaired.

PROS AND CONS OF JUICING

As with everything in life, juicing too has unique benefits and notable drawbacks. Given how important a change can be to start an entirely new life habit, it's important that you're properly educated about all the dimensions of juicing. Here are the most common pros and cons of juicing (Mather, 2014):

+ Pros

The benefits of juicing are vast. First and foremost, juicing provides a solution for some of your biggest problems, like getting enough nutrients without investing too much time in cooking and food prep. Aside from being a great method to consider nutrients, here are more pros to taking up juicing:

Extra Fruits and Vegetables in Your Diet

Vegetables are often made as side dishes to meat and pasta, meaning that we don't get nearly as much nutrition as needed from them. For those who don't like eating vegetables, juicing is a clever hack to have all the nutritional benefits without having to eat what you don't like.

Lean Nutrients

Quality juicers extract the beneficial nutrients from your fruits and vegetables, leaving the extra pulp that helps control blood sugar. The juice is then easily absorbed into your body and reaches your cells and tissue quickly and easily.

Nutrient Preservation

Many precious nutrients are heat-sensitive. They're essentially destroyed during cooking. Juicing doesn't only get you out of eating veggies. It provides you with many minerals, phyto minerals, and vitamins that would otherwise be lost with regular cooking.

Balances Acidity

Your usual diet contains foods that form acids, such as meat, alcohol, sugar, and white flour. These acids are fed into your cells. Researchers have discovered that acidity has been associated with life-threatening illnesses. Juices introduce a balancing, alkaline influence to your diet by introducing more alkaline foods, like vegetables.

Improves Nutrient Absorption

The long years of eating on the go can affect your body's ability to absorb nutrients. You may eat a healthy diet, but your body still doesn't get all of the nutrients because your digestion gets impaired. Juicing produces nutrients that are effortless for your digestive system to absorb. Plus, many of the micronutrients in veggie and fruit juices are prebiotics. They serve as food to your gut microbiome and help replenish the intestinal flora so that it can keep performing its protective role.

Supports Immune Health

Did you know that juicing can help prevent allergies and numerous chronic illnesses? Modern life imposes exposure to toxins in the air, and chemicals are found all around you–in food, water, skincare, and other products you're using. These harmful toxins can hurt your immune system and make you chronically ill. A boost of nutrients from your juice can strengthen your immune system and help prevent chronic illness.

Better Look

As your cells replenish, your skin and hair begin to glow. You won't only look fresh, well-rested, and rejuvenated, but you'll also lose weight more efficiently. It also helps improve exercise performance.

Quick Energy Boost

One glass of nutrient-dense juice in the morning, and you'll feel amazing! Take it on an empty stomach, and you'll notice how your mood, energy levels, focus, and health improve gradually. Plus, all the additional micronutrients rejuvenate your cells and prevent premature aging.

Family-Friendly

Juices aren't yet another fad that only you can use. You don't have to hide them from kids or prepare them separately from the rest of your meals. You can serve your juices to kids and teach them how delicious healthy foods are, early on.

— Cons

There are some downsides to juicing that you should be aware of to get the most out of your new, delicious practice:

Lack of Fiber

Fiber is beneficial, both for health and weight loss. Yet, many juicers remove it by removing the pulp. Keep in mind that you can get a juicer that allows you to control if and how much pulp you want in your juice. Aside from adding the pulp to your juice, you can use it in many amazing dishes, which you'll learn later in the book.

Invisible Calories

Juices are so delicious that you can easily lose sight of the number of calories and amount of sugar and carbs that you're taking. It only takes a few extra calories each day, and you can start gaining weight without even realizing it.

Nutrient Imbalance

In this book, you'll be given a thorough insight into the best fruits for juicing as well as their nutritional values. However, juicing without proper insight into nutritional value can cause the excess of some nutrients on the one hand, and deficiency of others on the other hand. For example, if you drink a lot of juice during the day, some of the ingredients may suppress your appetite. You may eat less of other beneficial foods and begin to lack protein or fat. Additionally, drinking juice without insight into which nutrients you lack may prolong your nutrient deficiencies. You simply might not be using the right foods for juicing, and missing out on the opportunity to repair nutrient deficiencies. At the same time, you might get an excess of nutrients that are found in large quantities. When it comes to fruits and vegetables, this would include vitamin C, magnesium, calcium, and other commonly known nutrients. This is one of the major reasons why so much attention in this book is given to nutritional values.

THE COMMON JUICING METHODS

Have you noticed a surge of juice bars in your town? Perhaps, a juicer became a household item for many of your friends and acquaintances, and you're now wondering where the trend came from. In part, it's because the benefits of juicing have been long established, which created an increased demand. Yet, the bigger part of why juicing became so popular is that it became more accessible over time. Only a decade ago, you didn't have much choice regarding your juicer. Perhaps, you could choose its capacity in terms of bowl and auger size, but brands varied when it came to the potency of juicing. Yet, the process of juicing used to be very exhausting, so it's no wonder that only people willing to invest time and effort into it got their juicers. Juicing required a lot of fruit, much of which ended up getting thrown out.

Nowadays, the production of juicers has significantly advanced. Manufacturers pay attention to the quality of materials and are now massively producing BPA-free juicers. The apparatus itself became highly personable and less wasteful. You can choose speeds, modes, and many other options to optimize juicing. This, of course, doesn't depend on how fast you wish to produce your juice. You can choose various juicer settings based on the foods you're using, and adjust the settings to preserve maximum nutrients. You can choose how much pulp you want in your juice as well, which greatly affects people's satisfaction with juicing.

Now, the foods available for juicing are numerous. You don't have to do much but shop for your favorite fruits and veggies and get some convenient recipes. Yet, it's the selection of your juicer that affects whether it will serve your specific purpose. Are you looking to reduce sugar intake while maintaining the variety of fruits and veggies used? You have an option! Do you wish to make more sugary, energizing juices to support high-intensity training? That's possible too!

No juicer is one-size-fits-all. Your selection of apparatus to use affects the ease of preparation and nutritional values of your juices, which, in turn, affects your satisfaction and the results that you'll get from juicing. Now, you might have heard about people who weren't satisfied with juicing. That could well be attributed to taking a random approach of buying the cheapest, closest juicer and throwing in whatever leftover fruits and veggies they had lying around in their kitchen. In this book, you'll learn about everything that goes into successful juicing–from selecting the right machine to choosing the right ingredients. That way, you'll get the nutrition you need without unnecessary spending and food waste.

The first thing to distinguish when choosing your juicer is whether you want a centrifugal or a cold-press machine. Here are the basic features, pros, and cons of both (Brown, 2019):

Centrifugal Juicing

Traditional juicers, in plain words, grind a fruit or a veggie and separate the juice from the pulp using a strainer. It's pretty much a mechanical version of what you're able to do with your own hands, only easier and faster. Centrifugal juicers are more economical options. You can find a cheap juicer in the nearest store, and you don't have to spend a lot of time learning about different functions, features, and functionalities. You can use your centrifugal juicer to produce a lot of juice quickly, which makes these types of juicers the most popular and most common. With that in mind, here are some pros and cons of these juicers:

✚ Pros

Time-Efficient

Centrifugal juicers are quite powerful, and they go through a lot of juice within a short period. This makes them a great choice for a household that juices each day, with several people needing their juice supplies multiple times a day.

Family-Friendly

Given that centrifugal juicers enable quick prep, they're suitable for more purposes than just making juice for yourself. You can use them to make juices for children of various ages, and even sauces and condiments for other cooking. If you're looking to invest in a quality juicer, but you don't want it to serve the single purpose of making your juice, this is a great option.

Versatile

You can use centrifugal juicers on almost all fruits and vegetables. Their high capacity enables them to process thicker, harder fruits and vegetables quickly and easily.

Easy-Maintenance

A centrifugal juicer is as simple as it is versatile. As such, it's easily washed and serviced if needed. While there are variations in specifications, these machines generally operate using the same simple mechanism. This means that you'll have a much easier time keeping your juicer clean, and if needed, getting it fixed will be a lot easier and cheaper.

— Cons

Noise

As much as you can use your centrifugal juicer to prepare a tasty treat for a toddler or young child, you better not do it while they nap! Centrifugal juicers are known to be noisy, which can be inconvenient if you wish to make your juice early in the morning or you're using a device when other members of the household need silence.

More Waste

Centrifugal juicers use the simple method of cutting up foods using blades, but their mechanism for squeezing out the juice from the pulp isn't as refined as it is with a cold-press juicer. This means you'll be using more food with less juice as a result than you would if you used a cold press juicer.

Less Nutrient Preservation

Some nutrients break down with this particular technology. While cutting foods, a centrifugal juicer produces heat. This can negatively affect the quality of your juice, although you'll still have sufficient nutrients left in your juice for a quality drink.

Higher Oxidation

Many vitamins and minerals quickly oxidize when exposed to air. Centrifugal juicers allow air to penetrate the auger, which may cause oxidation faster than a cold-press juicer. Still, many users debate whether or not such a small level of oxidation is even relevant to consider in the big picture of juicing.

Cold-Press Juicing

At its core, juicing is a process in which the machine crushes the food to extract the juice. With some fruits and vegetables (mainly those that contain plenty of water), juicing is easy. You can squeeze an orange or lemon without the help of technology. But, what about spinach or rutabaga? It takes some fine machinery to squeeze and crush these foods in such a way as to get the most juice out, minimize waste, and maintain a rich taste of the juice.

A cold-press juicer extracts juice without using heat, which preserves the nutrients and hence, improves the quality of the juice. Yet, the quality of the juice you're getting comes at a cost. This juicer uses a hydraulic press, which makes the process longer-lasting and more laborious compared to a centrifugal juicer. With this in mind, here are some advantages and downsides to this method of juicing:

+ Pros

Nutrient Preservation

Since the juice is extracted by crushing food rather than grinding/cutting it, more nutrients are preserved. Additionally, the cold-press juicer doesn't produce heat, which further preserves the quality of your juice.

No Oxidation

Cold-press juicers don't allow air inside the auger, thus preventing oxidation while your juice is being prepared.

Better-Quality Juice

Cold-press juicers are said to produce better quality juice for several reasons. They preserve more nutrients and prevent oxidation. Aside from that, these juicers extract more liquid from the food. The juice comes out with a stronger flavor and is more saturated compared to the one from a centrifugal juicer.

Less Food Waste

Your cold-press juicer extracts more liquid matter from the foods, thus leaving you with less food waste.

— Cons

Longer Prep Time

Since the cold-press juicer crushes rather than grinding fruits and vegetables, it takes longer to produce juice. Essentially, working with this juicer means that you'll invest more time in a higher-quality beverage.

Higher Maintenance

Cold-press juicers require a bit more care in comparison to centrifugal ones. To get the most out of them, you need to think more about how much food you're adding to the juicer and how you combine foods. If your juicer breaks, getting it fixed will likely take a bit more time and money.

In this chapter, you learned about what juicing is, what types of juicers there are, what the pros and cons of juicing are, and other relevant must-knows. You learned that juicing can be a great way to boost your health and improve nutrition without having to eat more fruits and vegetables. Furthermore, juicing is an amazing way to enrich your diet without having to spend extra time cooking and eating. Within a single glass of juice, you can drink an entire meal's worth of micronutrients.

But, what about shortcomings? As you learned in this chapter, not understanding what juicing is and neglecting to pay attention to nutritional values can lead to nutrient deficiencies. Insight into your recommended daily calorie intake, as well as health and any potential nutrient deficiencies is essential for juicing to yield the much-needed result.

Now that you know more about the basics of juicing, it's time to learn a bit more about fruits, vegetables, and herbs that are known to be a great choice for juicing. This is necessary because too many people make grave errors with choosing random ingredients. With juicing, it's essential that you choose the ingredients that have the right nutritional benefits. It's also important that you combine the foods with educated insight into how certain tastes and nutrients work together so that you can better support your health. In the next chapter, you'll learn about the specific fruits, vegetables, and herbs that are best used for juicing. With this knowledge, you'll have easy access to shopping ideas, and a clearer image of the ingredients that you should use in order to achieve the results you're hoping for.

2

THE STAR INGREDIENTS

At the beginning of this book, I touched on the highly individual nature of juicing. Aside from getting the right juicer, your health and shape also rely on the choice of the right foods. Perhaps, you've heard some great misconceptions about juicing–that juices contain an unreasonable amount of sugar, and that going overboard will hurt your health. This couldn't be further from the truth! Here's a simple fact: fruits and vegetables have different nutritional values. Some have more carbs and sugars, while others pride themselves in the richness of fat and protein. You have an enormous range of foods at your disposal to entirely control how much of each macronutrient you wish to take with juicing. In this chapter, you'll learn about the best ingredients for juicing. These ingredients, which include fruits, vegetables, and herbs, are nutrient-packed and diet-friendly. Combine them carefully, and your magic potion will contain just the right nutrients for your needs.

BEST VEGETABLES FOR JUICING

Despite general belief, fruits shouldn't be your immediate go-to for juicing. In fact, this book will put more emphasis on veggies than fruits for several of the following important reasons (Link, 2019):

- Sugar control

Vegetables can be as tasty as fruits, but with much less sugar than you'd anticipate. Vegetable juices often have between 50 and 70 calories, meaning that they don't add too much weight (pun intended) to your daily means. It's important to understand that vegetable juicing is found to benefit health much more than fruit juicing.

- Nutrient density

Vegetables, in fact, have an equal amount of nutritional value to fruits, if not greater. Vegetables are better nutrition choices since you can pack a lot of nutrients in a single glass without many carbs and sugars.

- Diet composition

Nutritional recommendations mandate eating twice as many vegetables than they do fruits. In many ways, veggies are much more valuable for the body, but a lot less consumed since so many people dislike their taste. As opposed to fruits, whose single serving during the day settles for an average person's nutritional needs, we need vegetables as a side dish to all of our meals. For those who don't like eating vegetables, juicing is a neat cheat.

- Flavor

Vegetables lose a lot of flavor when being cooked, and most people are just not comfortable eating them raw. Juicing allows you to enjoy a unique vegetable flavor with the maximum of nutrients.

With this in mind, here are the best, most nutritionally valuable vegetables that you can use for juicing:

#1: Kale

Kale may not be the most popular vegetable when cooked, since making it so that it doesn't taste bitter takes effort. Squeezed kale, on the other hand, tastes a lot better. Not only does it add freshness to your juice, but it also gives it a boost of antioxidants. Antioxidants protect your cellular health and combat free radicals, which reduces the risk of cardiac disease, high cholesterol, cancer, and many other diseases. Kale also contains beta-carotene, as well as vitamins K, C, and A.

#2: Carrots

Carrots are among the most commonly used vegetables, and also the most misused. Although they contain an abundance of potassium, biotin, vitamin A, and pigments known as carotenoids, these nutrients most often don't get absorbed in sufficient amounts. This is mostly because cooking, and high temperatures in general, deplete the nutrients, and a big part of the nutrients that survive get extracted into the water, or just end up at the bottom of your cooking dish. Luckily, juicing gives you the ability to enjoy the fullness of carrots' nutritional potency. Plus, carrots work great with almost all other fruits and vegetables. You'll enjoy them with apples, ginger, greens, lemons, and others.

#3: Beets

Beets aren't only intense in color, but also nutrition. They have a delicious flavor that fuels your body with folate, manganese, nitrates, and potassium, all of which have amazing health benefits. One important thing to note is that beet juice gives you the nutrition you need daily, which usually comes from starchy food. If you're reducing or avoiding carbs, beet juice will be a great substitute. An even better trait of these royal-colored veggies is their neutral flavor, which goes great with almost all other fruits and vegetables.

#4: Cabbage

You're likely used to eating cabbage in the form of a salad or cooked dishes. Indeed, cabbage is packed with vitamins–mainly B6, C, and K. It's also tasty and goes great with citruses, beets, apples, carrots, and other vegetables. Juicing this vegetable will add doses of valuable nutrients, albeit with a somewhat sweet flavor. Having a little bit of cabbage regularly is said to boost your immune system, help regulate blood sugar, and reduce the risk of heart disease.

#5: *Spinach*

Spinach is a well-known superfood. It contains plenty of vitamins C and A, plus copious amounts of antioxidants, including lutein, kaempferol, and quercetin. Adding spinach to your juice helps regulate your blood pressure and reduce the risk of heart disease. It also helps you alleviate acid reflux. Since it can taste a bit bitter, it's recommended to combine it with otherwise sweet veggies, fruits, and citruses.

#6: *Broccoli*

Another childhood nightmare, broccoli is a healthy veggie that's an acquired taste. It has a distinct flavor, and many people dislike it despite knowing about its major health benefits. Broccoli is rich in numerous essential micronutrients, including vitamins C, A, and B6. Plus, broccoli contains plenty of potassium, a nutrient of great relevance for those looking to get fit or exercise.

Isn't it amazing just how many veggies you'd no longer have to cook by juicing? Eating these vegetables in the form of juice would give you all the nutrition you were hoping for, and in a much more pleasant experience. However, most vegetables, when juiced, have either a savory or a slightly earthy flavor. In juicing, it's important to balance the flavors carefully so that your juice is neither too sweet nor too savory. For that reason, the next section will show you the best fruits to pop into your juicer.

BEST FRUITS FOR JUICING

Feeling like adding some juicy sweetness to the mix? While no fruit's considered a bad choice to pop into your juicer, some fruits admittedly bring more flavor and nutrition to the table. In this section, I'll suggest some of the most versatile fruits to add to your daily juices. When mixing fruits and vegetables, it's important to get the taste just right. You'll notice that this list includes many fruits that you can successfully pair with leafy greens, carrots, and your favorite cruciferous veggies to achieve a delicious-tasting juice.

Here's a list of the best fruits to pop in your juicer (Wells, 2019):

#1: Apples

Apples are one of the most universal and widely known fruits. Their flavor successfully finds its way into pieces and even pot roasts when you're feeling adventurous. Yes, apples will also work wonders in the form of juice. You can drink pure apple juice, or mix it in with some spinach, kale, carrots, and lemon for extra nutrition. Aside from healthy fiber, apples have anti-inflammatory properties. They'll also help you battle allergies. However, keep in mind that apples contain a lot of sugar and carbs. Account for their nutritional values when adding them to juice. Another important thing to mention is that apples oxidize pretty quickly, no matter which juicer you're using. Pop them in right after chopping, and don't wait too long before you drink your juice.

#2: Oranges

Another common fruit that pleases the palate while introducing abundant amounts of Vitamin C are oranges. Oranges are widely known and used not only for juice, but also for salad toppings, sauces, and dips. Some recipes even pair them with poultry meat for a more exotic flavor. Adding oranges to your juice will help support your immune system. However, there can be some differences when it comes to flavor, sweetness, and acidity depending on the variety of your orange. Before purchasing the fruit for your juicer, check which variety they are and what you can expect in terms of flavor.

#3: Grapes

Grapes may not be as popular of a fruit as apples or oranges, but they sure are valuable. Similar to oranges, they consist mainly of water. You'll be able to make grape juice with very little waste. Aside from being delicious, grapes also help with controlling your cholesterol. They can help reduce risks of cardiac disease by reducing blood clots, and they also help with regulating blood sugar. Isn't it amazing to finally discover a fruit that doesn't make you dread excess sugars and carbs? One thing to be wary of when juicing grapes is whether or not you wish to add seeds. If chopped in your juice, seeds will add a spicy flavor, so your juice loses a bit of its natural sweetness. If you don't want seeds in your juice, you'll have to remove them manually.

#4: Pomegranates

With a richness of antioxidants that help prevent heart disease, arthritis, alzheimer's, and cancer, it's no wonder that doctors recommend this fruit. You'll love adding pomegranates to your juice since they're sweet but mild, and your juice won't taste overly sweet. However, it could take you some time to peel them. If you're adding pomegranates to your juice, make sure to peel and chop them beforehand. You don't want your other precious fruits and veggies just sitting there and oxidizing while you struggle to get your pomegranate out of its shell, right?

#5: Blueberries

These delicious berries are extremely juicer-friendly. They leave very little waste and have a nicely balanced flavor that dances between sweet and savory. If you're not entirely up for a sweet juice and you wish to spice it up a bit, add blueberries! Aside from being delicious, blueberries also have plenty of Vitamin B and they host a richness of antioxidants. Adding them to your juice daily will slow down aging and help reduce the risks of some of the most life-threatening illnesses, like cancer. There is, however, one downside to making blueberry juice. You'll need quite a bit of them for a glass of juice. Unless you wish to purchase a couple of packages for only one juice serving, feel free to pair them with other fruits and sweet-tasting veggies, like carrots and beets.

#6: Pineapples

If you were looking for a superfood that can help support muscle healing, pineapple will be a good friend. Pineapples are the only known food that helps promote muscle healing, thanks to a substance called bromelain. Otherwise, pineapples are rich in manganese and Vitamin C. Yes, they do have a ton of sugars and carbs, and yet, they taste extremely sweet. However, pineapples can be a great ally if you're working out or doing high-intensity interval training. They'll help your muscles recover quicker and help get you back up and running should your muscles need some loving kindness.

#7: Peaches

These yummy, juicy fruits are best in the late summer. Don't rush to pop them in your juicer, though. If you try to juice peaches before they're ripe, you might not get as much juice out of them as you hoped. Plus, they might also taste a bit savory. Let your peaches ripen in the sun first by letting them soften for a couple of days at room temperature. This way, you'll get a fuller taste. Better than that, you'll intensify their antioxidant properties. Eating peaches regularly helps you reduce allergies. It also helps boost your appearance, as the fruit will help you achieve shinier, smoother-looking skin.

#8: Cranberries

Cranberries are extremely healthy. However, their taste, admittedly, isn't for everyone. If you don't like the tart taste of this fruit, you better combine them with other ingredients. You may not enjoy the flavor as much as you hoped, but you'll reap some of its precious antibacterial properties. Cranberries contain antioxidants that help battle the bacteria that cause infections in your urinary tract. It also helps reduce LDL cholesterol, and overall boosts your immune system. However, this fruit may interact with certain medications. This is due to its potency, which further attests to its awesomeness. If you're adding cranberries to your juice daily, don't forget to first consult your doctor!

#9: Lemons

Surprised to find one of the most common juicing fruits almost at the bottom of the list? That doesn't mean that lemons are any less valuable than other fruits. However, their high acidity entails that you should only use them in small quantities. You shouldn't even attempt to drink pure lemon juice, since this could hurt your mouth and stomach. However, lemon juice will work amazingly with almost any other juice! It's particularly popular with a mix of carrots, apples, and spinach. Make a light green smoothie, such that it will support your metabolism, digestion, immune system, and thyroid health. Another important benefit of lemon juice is that you don't have to use up the entire lemon at once. You can add only a little bit to your juicer and leave the rest to sit in the fridge for days. The juice won't oxidize or lose its flavor and nutrients!

#10: Mangoes

Last, but not least is this buttery fruit that's been all the hype recently. Mangoes are among the few fruits that are rich in fat, which made them suitable for various low-carb diet plans. So, why are they so great for juicing? Aside from a unique flavor, mangoes contain a ton of antioxidants that help balance your blood sugar. The nutrients found in mangoes also help reduce asthma and improve your eye health.

Isn't this list just delicious? Even better, you don't have to go to great lengths to obtain these fruits. You can find almost all of them in your nearest grocery store! A word of caution when it comes to shopping: be careful about the varieties of fruits that you're choosing. When it comes to fruit, there are dozens of different varieties on the market. The variety creates a difference when it comes to nutritional values, taste, and the amount of water found in a particular fruit. Likewise, when shopping, pay attention that your fruits are sufficiently ripe. Fruits that are too hard may prove hard to juice. To help your fruits become softer and more juicer-friendly, let them sit for a couple of days before using.

In this section, you learned about the wonderful fruits that you can add to your juice that can balance out the veggie flavors. Yet, there are more ways to improve the taste of your juice. In the next section, you'll learn about delicious herbs that you can add to your juice. As you're about to learn, herbs can make for a potent addition to your diet, and give you more rare nutrients without the cost of extra calories and sugar.

THE BEST HERBS FOR JUICING

Herbs aren't only nutritionally valuable. They add a special flavor to your juice and can make two juices made from the same fruits and vegetables taste completely different. You can use herbs to adjust the flavor of your juice to your liking and to enhance the nutritional value of your beverage. Herbs are quite nutrient-dense. They contain high amounts of vitamins and minerals. Some of that nutrient density can be attributed to the fact that we consume herbs in dehydrated form. That way, herbs, and spices become more potent since a high amount of nutrients is condensed in a small quantity of food.

Aside from achieving a richer juice flavor, herbs are beneficial as they have anti-inflammatory properties. These properties protect your immune health and strengthen the performance of your immune system. Antioxidants also help prevent numerous chronic and life-threatening illnesses.

If you were looking to add a special note to your juice, you should try the following herbs (Juicing Herbs, n.d.):

#1: Basil

This popular herb tastes great whether dried or fresh. It has a unique scent and will add gentle freshness to your juice. More importantly, it goes great with the majority of vegetables–especially leafy greens, as well as apples, lemons, and other citruses. If you use basil in your juices, you will enrich your beverage with an abundance of Vitamin C, A, and K. It also contains calcium, omega 3s, and magnesium.

Aside from supporting immune health, basil also contributes to reducing infections and inflammation.

#2: Mint

The unique mint taste is recognizable no matter the type of food and beverage. You won't need a lot of it for delicious juice! Although mint works best with leafy greens, when combined with citruses and apples; it will produce one of the most memorable drinks you have tried so far. This combo is even better with pineapple. If you were looking for a treat and delicious beverage that doesn't include alcohol, just add a bit of mint to your drinks.

#2: Oregano

You'll most likely see oregano sprinkled over a pizza or added to pasta toppings. This herb adds a bitter flavor to the dish, although still refreshing. It can be strong and overpowering, so make sure to only add a pinch to your juice. You might think that a herb like oregano doesn't belong in juice, yet it will work wonders for any juice that includes tomatoes, apples, or oranges. This herb works great with all products that taste bitter-sweet or have a savory note to them. Given the richness of antioxidants and Vitamin B in this plant, you wouldn't want to miss out on it. However, if you wish to conceal its strong flavor, you can do so by combining it with a little bit of ginger.

#3: Parsley

Commonly used in soups, stews, and pot roasts, parsley is one of the oldest herbs to find its way into an average kitchen. Not without a reason though, since it contains a ton of micronutrients, from Vitamin C, K, and A, to potassium, magnesium, calcium, and iron. It doesn't have a neutral flavor though, so have some ginger by your side if you don't have a taste for the bitter note it adds to your juice. You'll mix parsley successfully with any juice that contains apples or carrots. The sweetness of these plants will additionally balance out the parsley, and result in a much better-tasting juice.

#4: Rosemary

Now, we come to one of our favorite Mediterranean herbs to add to all sorts of dishes, and in some cases, even sweets and pastries. Rosemary has a distinct smell and taste, and it adds exotic freshness to your juice. However, unlike other strong-flavored herbs, this one doesn't overwhelm and will work together with other produce to blend into a unique taste that will vary depending on the foods you add to your juicer. It will taste particularly nice with pears and limes though, and it will add a ton of copper, potassium, and vitamin B6 to your juice.

#5: Thyme

While the previous delicious herb contained rare copper, some thyme in your juice will pair this super nutrient with some extra zinc, thiamin, magnesium, and Vitamin E. Combined, these ingredients strengthen your immune system and help it become more resilient to bacteria and viruses. Even better, it has a soft flavor that won't overwhelm your juice or stand out too much. This makes it great for any kind of fruit or vegetable, especially when combined with ginger and beets. The subtle taste of this herb will also work wonders when combined with citruses, fruits, and carrots.

#6: Ginger

Ginger has a recognizable flavor that works great with fruits, vegetables, sweets, and even meat. If you want your juice to have a stronger, almost spicy flavor, you can amp up the ginger. However, if you add only a pinch, you'll get the gentle, refreshing note that most people like. Ginger contains a ton of vitamins, and is known to benefit metabolism as well. However, it is a root plant, meaning it doesn't contain a lot of liquid. Before juicing this delicious root, make sure to wash it and finely chop it. That way, your ginger will get squashed into the finest pieces while juicing, which will extract more juice.

#7: Fennel

Fennel contains a long list of minerals and vitamins. It will give you a boost of nutrition to support your heart and bone health, and it will also help control blood pressure. It contains a phytonutrient called anethole. This rare nutrient not only supports immune health, but it also helps protect your nerves, balance out blood sugar, and is also found to prevent cancer and leukemia. The mild flavor of this herb will remind you of licorice, and you'll easily mix it with other fruits and vegetables.

#8: Chamomile

A pinch of chamomile with your fruits and veggies will add a warm, nourishing note to your juice. Beyond that, chamomile has proven benefits for immune health and preventing chronic diseases. This includes heart disease and cancer! You don't need a lot of chamomile in your juice though, since only a pinch will suffice to boost the flavor. Keep in mind that increasing the amount of chamomile in your juice won't necessarily intensify the flavor. Once the juice is saturated and there's not much water left for the chamomile flavor to dissolve, the extra will simply go into pulp. You will have thrown out the majority of the help that you intended to use. Because of that, consider adding chamomile to juices made from otherwise watery plants.

#9: Nettle

Last, but not least, nettle has numerous nutritional benefits. It helps your kidneys and liver detox thanks to an abundance of vitamins and minerals. The herb itself tastes similar to plain spinach, only somewhat stronger. With that in mind, you can add it to any juice recipe that otherwise works well with spinach. Worried about the sting? You can relax. The plant's distinct property, in this case, doesn't extend to its juice.

Herbs can make each new glass of juice taste differently. You can use herbs to alter the flavor, and to also add specific nutrients to the juice that address the specific ailment that you wish to treat.

In this chapter, you learned about the best ingredients to use for juicing. Doesn't it surprise you that some of the more popular fruits and veggies aren't on the list? This is because in this book, I aimed to present you with ingredients that affect and benefit your health the most. Now, you have a simple shopping list that you can take with you to get the exact foods you want.

But, wait! Juicing is so much more than a list of foods. To make juice each day and to make this new practice effective and enjoyable, you'll need the right set of tools. For that reason, the next chapter will focus on the equipment needed for successful juicing.

3

LINING UP YOUR JUICING TOOLS

Have you ever seen a chef working in an ill-equipped kitchen? Food is a symphony of textures and flavors, yet we can only access its magic with the assistance of proper tools. The tools of the juicing craft are as relevant as the food itself. In the same way that one can't cook properly without a good stove, dishes, and utensils; one can't make juice without the proper equipment. In this chapter, you'll learn the nuances of juicing tools, their proper use, and correct maintenance that will extend their lifespan and make your investment worthwhile.

Now that you know how to stock your kitchen for some delicious juicing, let's go over the equipment and tools that you'll need.

With the right tools, your juice will have maximum nutrition and freshness. They'll stay like that for a long time. The first step, of course, is to find the right foods. You know which veggies, fruits, and herbs you have at your disposal, and you can discover dozens of delicious recipes that serve your purpose. The second step in successful juicing is washing and prep. Give your foods a thorough wash, and make sure that they're all peeled and chopped for the kind of juice that you're making.

At this stage, you'll need a careful choice of equipment, starting at prep tools and your juicer. Your choice of juicer may affect how your juice will taste, how long it will last, and how nutritious it will be.

THE JUICING EQUIPMENT

To start with, you first need to choose between a centrifugal, masticating, and citrus juicer. Each of these juicers has unique advantages and disadvantages. Given that these different types of juicers affect your entire juicing process, let's review each type so that you can figure out which will work best for you (Treehuger, n.d.):

Centrifugal Juicer

These juicers are also called extractors. This is because they have a spinning blade that chops the produce directly and grinds it into juice. Although they tend to produce better quality juice, these juicers have many parts that you'll need to hand clean after each use. If you were relying on your dishwasher for all that work; sadly, it might not help. Dishwashers typically can't get all of the pulp out of a juicer, so you'll likely end up washing it by yourself either way. One major disadvantage of this juicer is that it produces heat while operating, which can kill off important, yet fragile vitamins and enzymes. Another important disadvantage of this type of juicer is that it becomes quickly oxygenated. As the juicer operates and spins its blade, a lot of oxygen penetrates inside and mixes in with your juice. Once your juice is exposed to oxygen, it needs to be consumed very quickly or else it may lose its nutritional value.

Masticating Juicer

As mentioned in the first chapter, the masticating juicer produces beverages of incredible quality and flavor. Juices from the masticating juicer have fuller color, they're more opaque, and have a more intense taste, which all attests to the fact that this juicer does a better job at getting all of the nutrients into the juice. That doesn't come without a price though. This juicer is incredibly slow, and it will take a lot of time for it to produce a glass of juice. However, it will squeeze your produce dry (literally) and leave mostly dry pulp, meaning that most of the product gets used up. The oxygen also doesn't penetrate the juice, which means that you won't have to drink all of it right away. You'll be able to store it in the fridge for up to a couple of days. The masticating juicer is also a bit more expensive compared to the centrifugal one.

Citrus Juicer

Are you intent on making citrus juice each day? Many people enjoy their daily glass of lemonade or a fresh glass of orange juice in the morning. If you wish to make a simple juice made from only a single citrus fruit, then perhaps you don't need an entire juicing apparatus. Plus, citrus juices are heavily diluted with water, so why spend so much time and electricity when you don't need to produce that much juice? In this case, you can use a citrus juicer. This simple kitchen tool is designed to easily remove citrus juice, without splatter and waste.

There are numerous types of citrus juicers, from manual ones to electric-operated apparatus. Juicers of this type also differ when it comes to size and power. Aside from being a great solution for quick citrus juice, these juicers also make for a great present, whether it be for a wedding, birthday, or anniversary.

When it comes to choosing the kind of juicer you want, pay attention to style and functionality, as well as the amount of juice that you'll likely be producing each day. Similar to other juicers, you don't need an overly potent machine for only a glass or two of juice. Buying a more powerful citrus juicer is only justified if you'll be making larger quantities.

DO'S AND DON'TS OF USING A JUICER

Like all machines, juicers have their way of functioning. They have distinct strengths and weaknesses, which you should know about to get the most use out of them. After all, you want to produce large quantities of delicious juice every day, ideally without having to re-purchase a machine every couple of months. You also want high-quality juice, which will contain maximum nutrients, and which will taste great. Yet, there are common mistakes that can both damage your juicer and reduce the quality of your juice. To prevent them, here's a short list of juicing do's and don'ts:

Juicing Do's

Keep up the hygiene. Your juicer must be thoroughly cleaned after each use. It won't be enough to just pop the parts into the dishwasher. Remove all the washable parts and wash them manually, while making sure that all chunks of food are removed.

Start slow and speed up slowly. This speed rule applies to blenders as well. Give each of the slower speeds a couple of seconds before moving on to the higher ones.

Stay safe. A juicer should never be plugged in while you're dismantling it. The obvious reason for that is that it has sharp blades that can cause injuries if the machine is switched on by accident.

Store juicers safely. Your juicer should ideally be kept in a cupboard, where the temperature is neither too high nor too low. Keeping your juicer someplace dark will ensure that strong daylight doesn't affect plastic and other sensitive parts. You should also make sure that you're keeping your juice someplace dry, so that moisture doesn't cause rust, corrosion, or mold/mildew.

Juicing Don'ts

Now that you know how to properly care for your juicer, you should also avoid doing the following in order to avoid compromising the quality of your juice and to prevent your juicer from breaking down:

Avoid using thick, dry foods. While some juicers are made to extract juice from pretty much everything, it can't be said for the majority of commonly sold brands. Most of the time, you'll need fruits and veggies with high water content. You can add dry ingredients for flavor though, like herbs and nuts.

Avoid causing damage to the auger and blades. While juicers can have very powerful augers and sharp blades, they can get blunt very quickly if you use too many hard items. This would include whole nuts, ice cubes, and other things.

Repair the juicer on your own. A juicer should only operate with the manufacturer's parts. If you try to repair the machine on your own and replace the parts, this could have catastrophic results. You could even cause a short fuse or a fire, putting yourself at risk. Make sure that only licensed professionals handle your appliance!

ESSENTIAL JUICING TOOLS FOR YOUR KITCHEN

Juicing is generally quite easy and clean, especially if you use one of the more modern juicers that operate faster. You won't need many tools aside from your juicer and produce. However, the few tools that are needed should be of high quality. The remaining tools more or less serve for food prep and juice storage, and aren't necessary for the juicing process itself. The good news is that you don't need any tools aside from those that you already have in your kitchen. Here are the tools needed for easy and successful juicing:

Knife

You'll need a quality knife for speedy and precise food chopping. Your knife must be sharp, first and foremost. You'll use it to peel, slice, mince, and cut your produce into exact pieces that are optimal for juicing. It's up to you whether you wish to have a whole set of knives just for juicing, or you wish to use one of the knives that you normally use for cooking. Whichever knife you pick, it should have a hard blade. Knives with thin blades get blunt very quickly, while those with hard blades tend to be more durable. Also, your knife should be resistant to corrosion. You'll be handling a lot of foods that contain strong acids, which could damage the knife over time. Ice-hardened steel is a great choice since this kind of knife is durable and will resist corrosion. You can also think about whether or not you wish your knife to remain sharp for a longer time, or you want a quality knife that's easy to clean and lasts a long time but will need frequent sharpening.

Cutting board

There's a variety of cutting boards available out there. You have plastic, wooden, ceramic, and many others. When it comes to juicing, you want a cutting board that's easy to keep clean. You don't necessarily need an expensive board, just one that will serve the specific purpose of being used to chop fruits and veggies. Most households have multiple cutting boards with different sizes, shapes, and materials that are used for different purposes. The size of your board depends on the quantity of food that you wish to prepare all at once. For juicing, the size of your board will depend on the average amount of produce that you wish to cut. So, if you're cooking a lot each day, you'll need a larger cutting board. If you're prepping a dish or two each week then a small board will do just fine. However, I advise using a separate cutting board for your juice. Boards can sometimes absorb smells from food, so your board can transfer bitter tastes that remain after cutting onions or meat. No matter how thoroughly you wash your board, these are hard to remove completely. Bamboo boards have been said to be more popular among people who juice than other materials. Bamboo is easily washable, and also light. Whichever board you choose, make sure that you can wash it thoroughly and that it's used specifically for juicing.

Cleaning brush

You'll need a quality brush to not only clean your juicer but also your cutting board and knife. Your brush can extend your juicer's life span by a considerable amount of time by preventing corrosion. You'll need a quality brush that can pull out pulp and food residue from pretty much every nook and cranny of your juicer. Considering that you can't fully rely on your dishwasher to complete the job, nor you can access all parts of the juicer with your sponge, a cleaning brush is the next logical choice. Cleaning your juicer with a brush each day will ensure that all bacteria and acidity from the machine are removed. That way, you'll know it's safe to drink your fresh juice, and your juicer will also last longer.

Apple and pineapple corer

A corer is a round tool that helps chop and core fruits and vegetables neatly. It is shaped like a round, hollow lever with a sharp bottom edge. Around the end of that lever, there's a round blade that cuts the "meat" of the fruit into a spiral. You core an apple by inserting the bottom of the tool into its core and then pushing the tool through the fruit. Once you pull the tool out, you're left with a hollow apple that you can later chop, or stuff and bake. With pineapples, a corer ensures quick and easy peeling and cutting. Upon cutting up the top and the bottom of the fruit, all you need to do is begin to twist the handle and allow the round plate to pierce its way into the meat of the fruit. The process is finished after the round blade pierces through the other side of the pineapple. You can then pull the tool and the pineapple meat out. You'll get a roll of spiral-shaped pineapple meat with a whole inside. You can either use the fruit as is or chop it up and add it to your juicer.

Vacuum juice containers

Vacuum containers are amazing because they allow you to pull all of the air out and protect your juice from oxidation. You can also find BPA-free containers. Vacuum containers don't only prevent oxidation and nutrient decay. They also keep your juice sanitary. Most bacteria and viruses can't survive and multiply without air. Still, be sure not to store your juice for over 72 hours. If you're using non-vacuum containers, like mason jars, your juice will stay fresh for no longer than 48 hours.

Peeler

Peelers are useful for fast food prep. The rules for purchasing quality peelers are similar to those for knives. The handle should be sturdy enough to endure pressure and pulling, while the blade needs to be sharp and rust-resistant. Splurging on a quality peeler might seem like a waste of money, but it's not. It will save you a lot of time during food prep, and you'll have more energy to think about adding a variety of foods and herbs to your juice.

TIPS FOR KEEPING YOUR JUICE FRESH FOR LONG

The rule of thumb when it comes to juicing is that you should have freshly made juice as often as you can spare the time. But, what if you don't have the time? What if you need your pre-made juices for those days when you can't spend time in your kitchen preparing fresh ones?

In that case, it's necessary to store your juice properly so that it doesn't spoil, oxidize, or lose all of its precious nutrients. Luckily for you, there are ways to store your juice in such a way as to preserve its freshness and nutrients for a couple of days. Follow these guidelines for storing juice, and you'll never run out of freshly made health drinks:

Keep juice at a maximum of 48-72-hour shelf life

With an exception of citrus, juices tend to not have a long shelf life. You may keep them unspoiled by refrigerating, but even then, you'd have to throw out your juice after four to five days. Even if the sugar inside your juice didn't cause it to ferment in the meantime, your juice will have lost the majority of its nutrient potency. All in all, account for storing the juice for no longer than two or three days. One way to ensure that you neither run out of pre-made juice nor make too much, is to carefully calculate how much juice your household drinks daily. If the quantity isn't regular (e.g. you and your family drink a lot of juice on some days and no juice on others), try and remember how much you have on average. That way, there's less chance of having to either throw out the extra juice or choose to drink more than recommended to avoid waste.

Choose what food to juice

Not all foods have an equal shelf life. Citruses, like lemons, limes, and oranges, are known to be long-lasting, whereas apple juice, for example, oxidizes within minutes in the fresh air. There's a simple way to tell how long your juice will last, and it's by the PH levels of the fruit or veggie. The lower the PH, the longer the juice lasts. But, there's another way to tell how long your juice will last. A rule applies here that says that acidic juices last longer, while sweet ones don't last as long. Your leafy greens and citruses can live up to the 72-mark, while your root plants and sweet fruits won't last for longer than a day. The reason for this is that the microorganisms, like bacteria and fungi, when allowed to grow in your juice in contact with oxygen, thrive in sweet environments. Fruit contains a lot of sugar, as well as root vegetables. As soon as bacteria and other microorganisms seed into the juice, they trigger the fermentation process that spoils the juice.

Use a slow juicer

Slow juicers, although a bit more laborious, still keep the air out of your juice. That way, they prevent oxidation and they also prevent the growth of microorganisms in your juice. The bacteria and fungi that normally inhabit each food that's exposed to air wouldn't be a health hazard if it wasn't for the generous quantities of sugar. Sugar is an ideal food for many of said microorganisms, so your juice becomes a fast-food stand for germs that are looking to feed, multiply, and thrive. You can block this process by preventing the air and microorganisms from entering your juice, and a slow juicer is the best machine to do that.

Filter to remove the pulp

Removing the pulp will make your juice last longer. The pulp is made from fiber or starch, which breaks down into sugar over time. Sadly, this process runs quickly with juices. When left inside your juice, the pulp will dissolve and not only spike the sugar inside your beverage, but also begin to feed the microorganisms mentioned earlier.

Add some natural preservatives

Many natural preservatives won't harm the nutrients in your juice. The first and most recommended is the addition of acidic foods. Acids, combined with Vitamin C, make it harder for bacteria and fungi to live and thrive in your juice. Aside from the citric acid, you can also add honey, malic acid, sodium benzoate, and potassium sorbate to your juice.

Store in vacuum-sealed airtight containers

Vacuum containers are accessible and simple to use. Most of them are made from sturdy, high-quality plastic, and feature a tool to extract the air from the bottle through its lid. Combined with a slow juicer, vacuum containers can completely rid your juice of contact with air, thus making it impossible for germs to thrive inside the beverage.

Use a dark or opaque container

Did you know that sunlight can destroy many nutrients in your juice? Vitamins and minerals from all over the alphabet are sensitive to sunlight. If not sunlight, they're extremely sensitive to heat. The more light that passes through the container, the greater the danger of your nutrients decaying; despite your best effort to preserve the juice. In particular, rare nutrients like Vitamin B complex and Vitamins A and D are very easily destroyed with sunlight exposure. If you're storing your juice in a refrigerator as recommended, it will be in the dark most of the time. However, you will expose the juice to sunlight whenever you open your refrigerator door, which could amount to significant time over several days. Get only opaque containers, and you'll preserve a lot more nutrients than you would in your regular jars.

Refrigerate

Vitamins and minerals quickly decay at room temperature, and germs find it extremely easy to inhabit the juice when it's not stored someplace cold. I wouldn't recommend keeping your juice in a kitchen cupboard or a pantry for that reason.

In this chapter, you learned about all the tools needed for successful juicing. From knives and cutting boards to juice containers, you now possess full insight into the instruments you need for spectacular juice artistry. You will use these instruments to carve, chop, squeeze, and safely store juice to preserve treasured nutrients and prevent all sorts of pesky microorganisms from inhabiting your beverage. Beyond hygiene and lifespan, the tools of the juicing trade enable you to smoothly make juice each day, without much hardship and mess. This is important for many reasons. If you want to juice for months, and even years at a time, you need to learn how to make the process easy and enjoyable.

Now that you know the juicing prerequisites, it's time to learn yet another important lesson about your juicing efforts. This lesson, summed up in the next chapter, is all about maximizing juicing benefits and results. In the next chapter, you'll learn about the three crucial steps of making quality juice. With this knowledge, you'll set yourself up for success with juicing, and more importantly make your time, effort, and resource investment worthwhile. Now, it's time for you to learn how to clean, prepare, and use up all of your juicing ingredients to the best of your ability.

4

GETTING THE BEST RESULTS

I f you thought that juicing was only about making and drinking juice every day, you couldn't be more wrong! In the previous chapter, you learned about all the tools needed to make quality, nutritious juice. However, much about experiencing the benefits of juicing also relates to how you clean and prep your juice and also what you choose to do with the remaining pulp. You see, each part of your fruit or veggie is nutritious. To miss out on the nutritional value would be such a waste, especially if it happened due to little mishaps in food cleaning and preparation. To start with, the next section will shed more light on the importance of cleaning your food properly before juicing, and the cleaning methods that efficiently remove dirt and germs without compromising the nutritional value of the food.

STEP 1: WASH YOUR FRUITS AND VEGGIES

Getting your foods all clean before juicing is essential for many reasons. Cleaning ensures that you not only remove potential toxins and germs from your juice but also help make the juice longer lasting. When pathogens are removed from your fruits and veggies, there's less chance that they'll find their way into the beverage and cause it to spoil faster than it usually would. Yet, most people only lightly rinse the food before the prep stage. Just rinsing the food, in this case, won't be enough.

The main reason for washing your fruits and veggies thoroughly before juicing is because you won't be cooking them. Cooking and frying typically kill off most of the germs, so you don't have to worry. But, with juicing, there's no high temperature to kill off the germs. Juicing is an entirely cold process in which liquid is extracted from food using physical pressure. Not only are all germs that come in contact with the liquid allowed to survive, but they're also kept extra fed by the high quantities of sugar found in the juice and pulp.

All in all, freshly squeezed juice is a fertile ground for all sorts of pathogens. Proper cleaning will remove said pathogens, debris, and toxins that are piled up on the surface of the fruits and veggies. Yet, there are several different cleaning methods that you can use to clean your food. Choosing the right method will preserve the food while adequately removing dirt and pathogens. In the next section, you'll find out which cleaning methods you can use, and which work better for certain foods than others.

Best Cleaning Methods

Traditionally, the most common way of cleaning food was by rinsing it with water. While this method can be successful, it is not always the best choice. Fruits and vegetables may lose quality if rinsed with water. Plus, some pathogens can remain on the surface of the food even though it has been rinsed with water. Rinsing alone likely won't remove all of the debris from the food. In some cases, it could make the matter even worse. For example, if your fruit or veggie still has traces of soil on it, and you wet it first, you'll create actual mud on your food. Such food will be hard to peel or cut without the mud getting inside it, after which removing the dirt becomes almost impossible. Here are additional ways to properly clean the food and remove any residual dirt or pathogens (Panoff, 2020):

Wiping/scraping the dirt off

If there's visible dirt and residue on your food, the best way to remove it before prepping is to use any dry cleaning method of your choice. Adding water before having scraped off the dirt will muddy up your food and potentially introduce dangerous pathogens and toxins to your juice. You can first use a knife or your hands to chunk off hard layers of dirt and soil from the food. Depending on the food that's being used, you can also use a dry sponge or a cleaning brush to scrape the dirt off more thoroughly. After that, you can grab a cloth and wipe the food clean before washing it. That way, once you get the food wet, you won't dissolve any toxins and dirt, which could potentially only cause them to soak deeper into the food.

Soaking in baking soda

Baking soda has been said to successfully extract dirt and toxins from food. Look it up online, and you'll see videos and images of food soaked in baking soda with layers of what appear to be dirt, foam, and gunk. While there's only loose evidence that baking soda contributes to more thorough food cleaning, it is possible that it helps remove finer dirt and debris that's otherwise hard to remove with water. This is especially important with foods that you can't peel, like cruciferous vegetables. These veggies are quite hard to wash thoroughly, but they still can collect and absorb quite a bit of dirt as they're exposed to air and elements. To soak food in baking soda, you should add a teaspoon of the powder for every two glasses of water.

Using electrolyzed water

There's also some scientific confirmation that water enriched with electrolytes might help to better clean your food. Although the evidence isn't as strong as you'd hope, it is still an additional option worth trying.

Avoid using produce washes or vinegar, as these weren't shown to significantly contribute to making your food cleaner. Other substances might be harmful or even lethal, like bleach and other chemical cleaners.

Washing Fruits and Vegetables With Water

Although there are additional steps that you should take in order to clean your food properly, washing it with cool water is still considered to be the best way of cleaning your food. According to many experts, you should only include other steps if needed. Below are some general recommendations for cleaning your food with water.

Wash only right before using. Getting fruits and veggies wet and leaving them damp in the fridge could create a fertile ground for germs, and speed up the decay of your food.

Make sure that your hands are clean. Sanitize your hands before touching your food. Any germs and other substances found on your hands can also enter your food and your juicer. Carefully wash your hands with soap and water, and then dry them thoroughly with a dry, clean cloth. This will reduce the chances of having any germs and pathogens from your hands transferred into the juice.

Cut out rotten or damaged parts of the food. If there's any bruising, stain, or rotting on your food, cut it out before washing and peeling. This will further prevent bacteria transfer.

When washing leafy greens and cruciferous vegetables, briefly soak them in water. The keyword here is "briefly." Many nutrients in your food are water soluble, and you might reduce the quality of your food if you allow it to stay submerged for too long.

As you can see, there are many ways to clean your food correctly without missing out on any of its vitamins, minerals, and fiber. Choosing the right cleaning method makes a crucial difference when it comes to the flavor and nutritional value of your juice. Proper cleaning is particularly important if you wish to use the skins when making your juice, as well as to avoid losing nutrients in the process of washing. Now that you know how to properly wash, scrub, and soak your veggies and fruits, it's time to learn a little bit more about quality food prep.

STEP 2: PREPARE INGREDIENTS FOR JUICING

If only juicing were as easy as popping ingredients into your juicer! Food preparation is a major item in all culinary ventures. To think that prepping your food matters less just because you're juicing and not cooking would be a grave mistake. You can enhance the flavor and the nutritional value of your juice with a little bit of learning about how to peel, chop, slice, and dice correctly. In this section, you'll learn how to prepare all of your ingredients for successful juicing. With this knowledge, you'll get the most nutritional value out of your food, and you'll also preserve your juicer. That's right! Improper food prep can reduce your juicer's life span, damage your auger or blades, and arguably make juicing unnecessarily messy.

If you ignored some general food-prep rules and carelessly added various fruits and vegetables into your juicer, you'd achieve one or both of the following:

- A poor-tasting juice with a ton of waste and pulp
- A broken juicer

Improper food prep before juicing doesn't only spoil your juice. It's not only the overly hard produce that can affect the juicer and produce less-than-desirable results. If you're overzealous with chopping and you add almost minced food to your machine, you'll lose out on many food benefits. Overly small pieces are much harder to squeeze, press, and chop, meaning that you don't benefit from finely chopping all produce either.

Instead, you benefit from peeling and cutting food in such a way as to secure maximum juice extraction with minimal food waste. Aside from the flavor, proper prepping will ensure an appetizing texture and longer shelf life for your juice.

For that, you should follow some general juicing prepping tips (Cross, n.d.):

- Make sure that your produce is as clean as possible. Considering that you're serving your juice uncooked and unpasteurized, you need to take reasonable precautions against germs and bacteria.
- Consider keeping the peel if you're certain that the produce is organic and high quality. The peel naturally contains a lot of vitamins and minerals. However, some health experts argue that plants that grow in polluted environments and are treated with harsh chemicals absorb some of that toxicity, and it's largely contained in the peel. It's a judgment call in any case. Still, whenever possible and if you think it to be safe, choose to keep your peel.
- Remove seeds whenever possible. Some fruits have quite tiny seeds, and picking them out can be drudgery. Still, make an effort to do it because seeds can make your juice taste more bitter or spicy. Account for your juice losing some of its natural sweetness if you choose to keep the seeds.
- Cut larger produce into quarters. Cutting large fruits and vegetables into overly small pieces doesn't only take time. The length of the process can contribute to oxidation and nutrient degradation. Unless your product is

extremely hard, the juicer should be able to take a bit larger chunks.

- If you wish to add products that are otherwise not juicer-friendly, you can do so by pureeing or blending beforehand. You can either add minced produce to the juicer or mix it with the finished juice for a unique texture and taste.

Here are some useful suggestions for preparing specific foods (Cross, n.d.):

Apples

Apples are, in general, juicer-friendly. If you want, you can core them, since the few seeds that they contain could affect the taste of your juice. You don't have to though, and instead you can either cut them into halves or quarters or simply pop in whole, unpeeled apples.

Beets

I like to peel the beet because I usually find traces of dirt that are impossible to thoroughly remove. Before peeling and chopping into quarters, you should also cut off the tops and bottoms of the plant.

Berries

There's no reason for any specific prepping when it comes to berries. However, they typically contain very little water, and trying to juice them will likely result in a lot of waste with very little juice. Instead, puree them and mix them in with the rest of the ingredients.

Carrots

Prepping carrots for juicing is the same as doing it for cooking. Cut off tops and bottoms, and lightly peel the surface of the plant to remove any dirt.

Cucumbers

Cleaning cucumbers and preparing them for juicing is done the same way as carrots. Cut the ends of the food and peel it. Some juicers might process the whole plant, while others will require you to cut it into halves, quarters, or weights–depending on the size of the food.

Citruses

You can consider adding the peel to the juicer. However, some experts advise that some substances in the peel could react with medications or fall heavy on your stomach, so consider carefully keeping the peel. If you don't want to keep the peel, cut off the ends of the fruit, and then manually peel it off. You can then cut the fruit into halves or quarters.

Papaya and Mango

It's very questionable whether or not you'd want to juice these fruits. They typically don't contain a lot of water, so you'll have to use a lot of food to get a little bit of juice. You can instead puree the fruit, and pop it in with the rest of your juice.

Melons

All types of melons should be cut, peeled, and deseeded. You'd do the same if you were making a fruit salad or prepping slices of fruit to eat, and the process for juicing isn't any different either. However, for successful juicing, you should also cut the fruits into slices and then cut each slice into halves, quarters, or eights.

Nuts

Add nuts to your juicer the same way you'd add them to any other dish. The shells must be removed, and you should keep the peel since it enhances the flavor.

Wow, isn't there so much to learn about juicing ingredient preparation? If you found this part of the process to be inspiring, you're far from wrong. Any effort put into learning how certain foods are best prepared for juicing is more than valuable. Food prep isn't a waste of time by any means. It can be fun, especially if you have all of the necessary tools lined up. You've now learned how to get your ingredients all prepped and ready to pop into the juicer. Let's say that your juicing process goes successfully, and you now relish in the glass after glass of opaque, flavored juice. What's next? There's one more thing to pay attention to, and it is how you use up your pulp. In the next section, you'll learn a bit more about proper pulp use and its importance.

STEP 3: USE THE LEFTOVER PULP

Remember how earlier, I said that each part of a fruit or vegetable is valuable and worth using? Your juice is a vital part of a healthy diet. To control carb and sugar intake, it is necessary to first separate the pulp. That way, you know that your juice isn't raising your blood sugar. But, wait. Why use extra fruit and vegetables for your other meals, and allow significant parts of the fruit you used for juicing to go to waste? Pressed or not, food is still food. Food is valuable, so we ought to respect it and use up as much of it as possible before moving on to fresh, new ingredients.

If you purchased a quality juicer, you'll be left with small amounts of well-pressed pulp. However, if you're juicing frequently, the pulp can amount to significant quantities that shouldn't just be thrown out. The pulp contains healthy fiber, peel, seeds, and other healthy parts of the plant that can be a beneficial addition to your diet.

Here's how you can use your pulp after juicing (Good-nature, 2020):

Composting

Composting is one of its most common uses for those who enjoy gardening. Anyone passionate about gardening is likely in constant pursuit of quality composting solutions. If you don't wish to use your pulp for any other purposes, this one will do just fine. Adding pulp to your gardening soil will improve its quality and will nourish your growing plants much better than industrial composting solutions.

Soups and broths

If you like soups and you enjoy making them, then you should try using your pulp to enhance the flavor of your warm dish. There are many recipes for pulp soups. Each is delicious and simple to make as long as it's done to your taste. Either way, the philosophy behind it is simple. Make any soup recipe that you like and pop in the remainder of the pulp from your juicer. However, do so last-minute, or preferably even after you've turned off the heat, in order to preserve as many nutrients as possible.

Pasta Sauces

It's equally easy to use your pulp for pasta sauces as it is to use it for any other dish. Typically, you can make the pasta sauce from pulp using ingredients that match or taste well with the original sauce recipe. For example, if you're making juice from leafy greens, apples, and citruses, you can add your pulp to create a delicious pesto sauce. On the other hand, if you've been juicing with tomatoes, berries, beets, and other similar plants, you can use this pulp to cook an amazing pasta bolognese, milanese, and other similar sauces.

Smoothies

You can add the pulp to your smoothies to make them thicker and enhance their flavor. Similar to making pasta sauces, the pulp flavors and ingredients should complement those of the smoothie.

Breakfast

If you enjoy a rich breakfast with a dose of veggies, but you don't want to spend time cooking, you can spice up the meal using juicer pulp.

You can add your pulp to omelets or even use it to make veggie burgers. You can also add the pulp to your favorite cracker recipe, or make some delicious guacamole or hummus.

Baked Goods

Pulp is a great addition to any of your favorite baked goods. If you're one among the many who know that baked goods should be avoided, but still can't help themselves from time to time; you now have a way to make your croissants and bagels more nutritious. Plus, if you're having a hard time getting your kids to eat veggies, there's a trick to get them to like healthy foods.

Add the juicer pulp to any of your favorite recipes for pastries and other baked goods. You won't only enhance the flavor, but you'll also add extra moisture to the delicious treats. If you add a bit more butter or olive oil, this will make a delicious alternative to your regular pastry.

For cupcakes, you can use the leftover pulp that contains ginger, apple, lemon, and carrot, and blend it into your recipe.

Popsicles

Your leftover pulp can also become a delicious treat. Popsicles are usually considered to be junk food because of their high sugar concentration. However, you can replace unhealthy ingredients with pulp that is left after you've made some delicious sweet fruity juices.

Clothing dye

Believe it or not, you can even dye your clothes using pulp from foods that contain strong pigments like beets, nettles, lavender, and others.

Fruit leather

Fruit leather is one of the easiest treats to make. All you need to do is grab some baking paper and line it with a little bit of oil or grease. Then, spread spoonfuls of pulp evenly across the plate and press them to create a thin layer. After that, the leather needs to dehydrate between 12 and 14 hours. It can later be cut into strips.

Cream cheese spread

All you need for this recipe is a little bit of cream cheese and pulp to mix with it. You can then top your veggie sandwiches or crackers with this delicious dip and enjoy!

Isn't it amazing what you can achieve with a little bit of effort? In this chapter, you learned about little steps that you can take to increase the value of your food and create better quality. You can preserve as many nutrients as possible while cleaning the food, and then ensure maximum flavor and nutrient density with proper juicing preparation. Finally, you can use the entirety of your fruits and veggies by finding alternate uses for the pulp. Without purchasing and eating extra food, you can add the pulp to your numerous dishes; from soups to pasta sauces, and even baked goods. Ultimately, if you don't find a proper use for your pulp, you can use it to compost your garden. Your plants will thank you!

Now, we come to the more practical part of your journey. It's time to collect your juicer, tools, and favorite foods from the list given in Chapter 2, and actually get to juicing.

However, a serious mistake that many juicing beginners make is adding ingredients to their juice randomly. Simply picking up food on a hunch about what's healthy and what you'll like the most isn't the best way to go about juicing. The art of juicing resides mainly in the recipes, which are as important as they are with cooking and baking. In the following chapters, you'll find awesome juice recipes, with the addition of food prep and juicing instructions. With these recipes, you'll create immersive flavors that will enrich your every day, planting a little bit of cheer into your life aside from the many vitamins and minerals that are seeded into your belly. Enjoy while making your juice!

5

JUICING FOR WEIGHT LOSS

There's an overall misconception that one would only gain weight by juicing, and that juicing is only recommended to fit people who are looking to build muscle. Juicing can be very supportive of weight loss. If you choose your foods carefully and emphasize those ingredients that contain plenty of protein and fiber versus carbs and sugar, you can contribute to strengthening your immune system, helping your muscles heal from intense exercise, and overall supporting cellular metabolism. All of this is crucial for fat burning.

A lot of the time, people think that juicing is bad for weight loss because drinking a lot of juice is tied to taking in a lot of carbs and sugars. However, we forget how difficult it is for the majority of people to eat enough fruits and vegetables and to replace all of those unhealthy carbs and processed sugars gained from white flour products, store-bought goods, sugary snacks, and drinks with healthy foods. Keeping up a healthy diet isn't easy. Most people who struggle with weight loss struggle with excluding unhealthy foods from their diet. In that regard, drinking natural juice, even if it contains plenty of sugars and carbs, is a healthier alternative to eating store-bought snacks and fast food.

Drinking plenty of juice for weight loss gives you the hydration and replenishing recovery power needed to keep up an intense exercise schedule in the long term. We mostly think of weight loss as a combination of dieting and exercise, and while doing so, we laser focus on the activities that are done daily. However, steady weight loss is a lifelong change in habits and routines. For many, it is the most difficult change since it involves controlling emotional appetite and regaining the ability to differentiate hunger from thirst and tiredness. Instead of just thinking about what you'll eat and drink in a day, you need dieting and exercising routines that can last for a month, three months, six months, and for some people, even up to several years.

The same rule applies to the evening when most people with obesity struggle to resist the urge to binge eat.

Evening hunger is much attributed to long-term weight gain. To a degree, it is a combination of mental and physical exhaustion combined with a hormonal imbalance stemming from being in a constant state of burnout. Anyone who has tried dieting knows that the most difficult part of becoming a healthy eater is resisting long evening meals while watching TV. What most people don't realize is that much of the agonizing evening appetite can be attributed to the sudden drop of insulin and blood sugar levels that result from an irregular eating, sleeping, and exercise pattern. While some can resist the urge and wait until morning, others start to feel genuinely sick unless they have a snack. What better snack to get your blood sugar just to the level your body needs, yet without the processed component that further damages your health, and with extra nutrients that help regain hormonal balance?

With this in mind, the following juice recipes will give you the exact nutrition that supports steady and healthy, fat burning.

HEALTHY GREEN JUICE

This image must sound familiar: a good-looking, fit person is waking up early in the morning and the first thing they do is pop a bunch of greens into a blender or a juicer and have their fill of healthy green juice. But, why is green juice so important for overall health and weight loss? First of all, green juice contains plenty of antioxidants. Antioxidants, as mentioned earlier, support a healthy immune system. Nutrients found in this green juice also support metabolism and prevent chronic and potentially fatal illnesses. Second, the antioxidants that are typically found in green juice help your body absorb nutrients. This is essential for people who struggle with obesity, since they typically have many other associated health issues like insulin resistance and other issues that keep them from absorbing all of the nutrients from their food.

Green juice is also high in chlorophyll and effective in reducing inflammation. However, you should avoid buying green juice, because it inevitably has far fewer nutrients compared to a homemade one. Here are the ingredients that you'll need for your green juice:

Ingredients

- Approximately five ounces of kale
- Three-quarters of a medium cucumber
- Two-thirds of a medium green apple
- Approximately two ounces of celery
- An ounce of lemon or a quarter of a medium lemon
- Half an ounce of ginger

Preparation

First, you need to wash your yummy produce and then–the prepping begins. Quarter your lemon while leaving the skin on and add it directly to the press. Next, add all of the remaining ingredients to your juicer and start pressing

Juicing Instructions

Want to make your green treat even healthier? Keep in mind that your juice shouldn't contain any yellow spots. Ideally, it will be dark green in color, and any other pigmentation might suggest that some of the ingredients are too ripe. To avoid this, it's essential to remove any ripe spots on your condiments before pressing.

Use as many peels from your products as possible, because some vegetable peels, particularly cucumber, contain a lot of vitamin D.

Equipment and Storage

For this juice, you'll need a quality cold-press juicer. You'll also need at least one quality knife, a cutting board, and a vacuum container shall you wish to store your juice. As always, this juice is best taken immediately. However, you can let it refrigerate as long as you drink it within 24 hours.

POWERHOUSE CABBAGE GREEN JUICE

With only 80 calories found within the 12 ounces of this amazing juice, this savory yet light recipe will keep you incredibly energized and provide a feeling of balanced energy throughout the day. It will only take about 15 minutes to prepare this juice. However, the health benefits of it will produce incredible results over time. Some of the benefits that this juice brings to the table include a ton of amino acids, preventing ulcers, and detoxifying the body while helping steady weight loss. This juice will also boost your immune system and help control blood pressure. The powerhouse juice also has plenty of vitamins K, A, and C, and it will help promote and improve your cardiovascular health, which is pretty important if you are trying to establish a more intense exercise or activity routine to combat obesity.

Ingredients

For this recipe, you will need:

- Two medium leaves of green cabbage
- About eight ounces of green apple
- Approximately two and a quarter ounces of chard or 11 and a half leaves

- About two ounces of kale or three-quarters of a cup
- One medium stalk of celery and one small lemon

Directions

Carefully remove all of the dirt from the produce. If you recall the advice from the earlier chapters, all the ingredients except for the lemon should be briefly soaked in water–but no longer than two to three minutes, since you want to avoid nutrients from the food being extracted into the water. Now, first place the lemon into the press and then add the remaining condiments or ingredients and begin grinding together and pressing the produce until your jug is full.

Juicing Tips

Allow the stems from your leafy greens to find their way into the press. They add plenty of flavor and consistency to your juice. As with the previous recipe, try to leave the peels.

If you dislike cabbage, you can swap the ingredients for the red alternative. Still, try to use the white chard, because any other variety (like red or rainbow chard) will give an unpleasant color to your juice.

Equipment and Storage

I'll always recommend drinking your juice right away. However, if you can't, you can leave it for up to a day in your refrigerator. Of course, the juice would have to be stored in your vacuum container. Other than that, a juicer and cutting equipment will suffice for this juice.

WATERMELON JUICE

This sweet beverage will add only 25 calories per glass of juice, and like the previous recipe, doesn't take longer than 15 minutes to prepare. This juice contains antioxidants and is also helpful with reducing inflammation, promoting skin health, supporting your cardiovascular health, fighting cancer, and profoundly hydrating your body to endure increased activity and speed up metabolism from intense exercise.

The ingredients needed for this juice are quite simple and straightforward. You need 15 ounces or three cups of cubed watermelon without seeds.

A fifth of lime will equate to one slice of lime and three to four mint leaves.

Directions

You shouldn't wash a carved-up watermelon if you've thoroughly removed its crust or shell. Insert the lime and the remaining ingredients into the press and begin preparing your juice.

Juicing Tips

Avoid overfilling your press so that you don't get an overflow of watermelon. Remember, watermelon has so much liquid that you can create the juice simply by pureeing it and even putting it inside a blender.

If you want to add a twist to your juice, you can insert a little bit of beets.

Since the watermelon skin contains nutrients as well, you can pop it into the juicer. However, keep in mind that this will slightly mellow the flavor of your juice.

Equipment and Storage

You'll need your juicer and tools for cutting–like a large knife and cutting board. Stick to your vacuum container, but drink your juice within 24 hours!

CLASSIC GREEN JUICE

This oldie but goodie is a very classic green juice that gives you potent nutrition with only 55 calories per glass. Keep in mind that this juice is more on the savory side, and its flavor may not suit everyone. However, drinking a glass of juice that you don't necessarily prefer is a small sacrifice to make, provided that you will reap the benefits of all of the protein and magnesium, folate, potassium, iron, and calcium that you'll receive. These nutrients will help prevent cancer, control your blood pressure, reduce inflammation, help weight loss, lower your cholesterol, and keep your blood sugar balanced.

The last of the benefits is the main one when it comes to weight loss. Balancing blood sugar is essential to get your cells to start metabolizing insulin and in turn, start burning fat. Without this process, your cells are starving for energy while the supplies in your fat cells continue to grow.

Ingredients

For this juice, you will need:

- One medium stalk of celery
- Six slices of ginger or half of an ounce
- Two-thirds of a medium green apple
- Four and a half cups of spinach
- A slice of a medium lemon
- 2/3 cup of chopped parsley
- Three cups of chopped romaine

Directions

As simple as it can be–simply wash all of the products and pop them in your juicer.

Juicing Tips

If possible, leave the peels on the apples and lemon, as well as the stems on your leafy greens. These parts are often discarded, but they contain an entire richness of nutrients.

You can control the sweetness of your juice by adding more apples, or a slice or two of pear. You can also make your juice more savory if you add more lemon beet juice.

This refreshing juice is quick and easy to make, and can also be done with a blender or a juicer, depending on how you like it better. If you are certain that your product hasn't been treated with dangerous chemicals, you can consider leaving the peels–this includes the beat as well.

Equipment and Storage

Aside from the basic juicing and prepping tools, you'll also need an apple corer if you wish to neatly core the apples. The ingredients in this juice will oxidize quickly, so make sure to have your juice the same day as when you made it.

LEMON AND GINGER GREEN JUICE

Another refreshing and savory juice that will give you a kick for an early start to the day is the lemon and ginger green juice! This recipe includes:

- Two whole lemons
- One stalk of parsley
- A cucumber
- A couple of apples
- An inch-long piece of ginger
- celery to your taste

This time around, you don't have to worry about food ratios and quantities. You can simply put as much of these foods as you like, and reduce the amount of the ingredients that you like less.

Instructions

First, wash all of your produce, and for this particular recipe, remove the peel from your lemons. All you need to do is pop them in your juicer and proceed with the process of juicing.

Juicing Tips

You can avoid using apples if you wish, however, you should substitute them for another ingredient.

You can add more lemon if you want your juice to be more savory. Or, you can increase the amount of cucumber if you want to achieve a more mild taste.

Although this juice can be stored for up to four days, you will ideally drink it right after juicing.

As with other recipes, I would recommend prepping your ingredients separately beforehand, and then storing them in your freezer.

Equipment and Storage

For this juice, you'll need a peeler if you wish to peel your produce neatly, aside from your juicer, knife, and board. Store your juice in a vacuum container!

ORANGE AND CARROT JUICE

This sweet, yet spicy juice is a great option either for an early morning or for a midday pick-me-up, because it will give you a subtle boost of sweetness that will energize you inside out. This juice supports your immune system and contains plenty of Vitamin C.

Carrots are known to benefit health across the board, while the swiss chard found in this recipe also has cancer-preventing properties.

Ingredients:

- An orange
- An inch of ginger
- One cup of carrots
- One lemon

Directions

The process of making this juice is simple and straight-forward. Wash, peel and cut your produce. Pop it into a juicer and add a quarter to half a cup of water if needed. Start juicing!

Juicing Tips

With this particular recipe, you don't have to obsess about how much of each ingredient you will need. The taste won't vary significantly if you include other ingredients like apples, celery, or cucumbers. This amazing juice has antibacterial and antioxidant properties, and it also contains polyphenols which help produce inflammation.

Equipment and Storage

Although greatly beneficial for your health, this juice shouldn't be left in the refrigerator for too long. Instead, aim to drink it within 24 hours. Don't forget to use your vacuum container! The equipment needed for this juice includes a cutting board, an all-mighty rust-resistant knife, and, as always, your juicer.

PARSLEY JUICE

A fun fact, parsley has been proven to support weight loss! Sadly, we don't use it in our cooking to the degree sufficient to reap all of the fat-burning benefits. Now, you can remedy this grave mistake.

Ingredients:

The basic ingredients needed for this juice are:

- One stalk of flat leaf parsley
- Some ginger to your taste
- One cucumber

Directions:

The prepping process is simple. You can also use a quarter of fresh lemon and an apple if you wish to add sweetness to the juice. If you don't want to use apples, you can instead swap them for a cup of diced cucumber. The steps for making this juice are the same as the remaining ones. Wash your produce and keep the skins if you wish. Cut the ingredients into halves or quarters, and cord the apple to prevent the seeds from adding bitterness to your juice.

EASY CELERY JUICE

Another powerful antioxidant and potent fat-burner; celery is known as a metabolic booster. Now, you're having it all juiced up in its unprecedented glory.

Ingredients:

- Two stalks of celery
- Two to three fresh limes

Instructions:

As the name suggests, you are to cut up your ingredients and chunk them into the juicer. Bon appetit!

Equipment and Storage

You can give this juice a bit more time than usual if you need it refrigerated in your vacuum container, but make sure to drink it within 48 hours. You only need a knife, a peeler, and a cutting board.

BEETROOT JUICE

This yummy juice sports an earthy flavor. Aside from helping you boost your metabolism, it will also energize you and support you in resisting the temptations of candy and snacks.

Ingredients:

- Two to three whole beets
- One apple
- One lemon
- One cucumber
- A stalk of parsley

Prepping:

Use your peeler to clean up the cucumber, beets, lemon, and apples, should you choose so. If you want to leave the peels, soak the food briefly in water.

Instructions:

Cut up your hard ingredients first, and then juice them as your machine requires. You can either add parsley to the juicer or mince it and add it to the finished juice.

Equipment and Storage

Beet juice is known to be long-lasting, similar to lemon. However, the apples in your juice will oxidize quickly. If you wish to extend the lifespan of your juice, add fewer apples. Aside from that, you can store the beet juice in your vacuum container for up to 24 hours.

WHAT CAN YOU EXPECT?

Juicing is a great supplement to your weight loss efforts. However, you need to keep in mind that juicing is not a diet. Juice cannot replace a meal. This is another common misconception about juicing, and a reason why so many people report having adverse effects from it. You shouldn't attempt to substitute your meals for juices, but instead make wholesome changes in your entire lifestyle, including exercise, daily habits, social habits, and diet.

Another common misconception about juicing is that you'll lose weight by substituting solid for liquid meals. This isn't true either. There's an exact calculation that each person can do when it comes to how many calories you should eat each day, and how many of them should come from protein, fat, and carbs/fiber. Your daily juices should fit into that calculation so that your net calories, net carbs, and net sugars don't go overboard.

So, you now must be wondering–why should you drink all of these juices if they don't directly support weight loss? The main reason behind juices benefiting weight loss lies in natural supplementation. Most of the time, we're unable to eat as many micronutrients as needed daily, and that nutrient deficiency affects immune functioning, hormonal balance, and metabolism. As mentioned at the beginning of this chapter, juicing has the role of supplementation on your weight loss journey. You'll only lose weight effectively if you instill proper eating and moving patterns.

So, let's briefly recap what juicing can do for your weight loss to notice visible results:

- Provide a satisfying treat so that you find it less difficult to resist candy and snacks
- Gives you an energy boost at the beginning of your day
- Help recover intestinal flora, which plays an important role in hormonal and weight regulation

JUICING FOR WEIGHT LOSS TIPS

Be mindful of your calorie intake. As with any other meal, juice can have a wide range of nutritive and caloric values and composition. Account for juice when planning your daily meals, because small daily changes can amount to significant ones over time.

Choose less sugary produce. You can have fresh juice each day and still avoid adding calories and sugars to your daily count. Choose from the list of the best ingredients given in this book, and you won't be mistaken!

Eat your pulp. You may not enjoy the pulp inside your juice, but make sure to use it up! Choose between pasta sauces, cheese dips, veggie burgers, and many other dishes that can only get tastier with extra fruits and veggies.

Mind your nutrition. Juices are an amazing nutrition supplement, but they can't make up for all of your nutrient needs throughout the day. Having juice doesn't mean that you shouldn't get your vitamins and minerals from other sources as well. This is particularly important if you're on a calorie-restriction diet. Calorie-restriction diets often lack zinc, Vitamin B12, iron, Vitamin D, and calcium. You'll have a really difficult time losing weight long-term if you lack these nutrients, given that they're linked with muscle regeneration, cardiac fat, and the functioning of your immune system. Make sure to choose those foods that compensate for the ones you're lacking in your diet.

Don't go overboard! You can have too much healthy food. It is possible to have too many vitamins and minerals from fruits and vegetables, which could put extra strain on your liver and kidneys. Only have the recommended amounts of juice, and drink to a degree that feels pleasant and comfortable.

Be extra mindful of infections. Drinking freshly squeezed nutrients each day increases your chances of catching an infection or inflammation. Write down clear rules for yourself, like washing your juicer each day, having juice immediately after making or storing exclusively in vacuum containers, drinking your juice within the adequate expiration time, and so on.

As you can see, juicing can be of great help for your weight loss. However, slimming down isn't the only reason why you should juice. After all, you may support fat burning with juicing, but what about getting rid of metabolic by-products?

In case you didn't know, your body's by-products are a notable part of what you perceive as excess weight. You might easily hold on to as much as nearly 10 lbs worth of liquid that your body struggles to eject. The reason for this is that your metabolic and physiological processes must work properly to eject the extra water and empty your colon to the degree needed for the body to continue properly absorbing nutrients. Furthermore, when your body is burdened by hormonal imbalance, insulin resistance, and slow digestion, all other beneficial processes slow down. Your nutrient absorption is depleted, and without it, your tissues and cells can't function properly. Some of the nutrients you eat do go directly into the blood, cells, and tissues, but another part of them is necessary to synthesize hormones and neurotransmitters needed to regulate your physiological processes, mood, and energy. This means that increasing nutrient intake alone won't necessarily heal all the damage that was done to your body's natural, physiological processes. These processes are being slowed down, if you will, in a mechanism similar to increasing speed while driving while simultaneously pressing your breaks. For these processes, which further speed up your metabolism and level up hormones, to function properly, it's necessary to support your body in ejecting metabolic products. As you're about to learn, this process isn't necessarily about stimulating urination and your digestive system. It's mainly about empowering your kidneys, liver, and glands to perform well under pressure. When this is done, your body has a much easier time getting rid of substances that are formed when you eat and burn fat.

The accurate process of doing so is called 'detoxing.'

But, wait, you've heard such terrible things about detoxing! You might have heard that detoxing is a fad, a sham if you will. That there's no reason to make an effort with detox, given that your kidneys and liver will do their job efficiently. What experts arguing for this fail to mention is that your liver, kidneys, spleen, glands, and other organs can suffer the same metabolic damage as the rest of your body.

In the next chapter, you'll learn how juicing can help you detox your body and get rid of toxic substances that are hurting your health. You'll also learn about the best juice recipes for detoxing, and of course, how to juice for detoxing correctly. With this information, you'll be able to estimate your detoxing needs and begin juicing in such ways that truly nurture and support your body inside-out.

6

JUICING FOR DETOX

R emember how we talked about damaged intestinal flora? Eat too many cheeseburgers and pizzas, and your stomach actually begins passing toxins from your food into the body. These toxins cause numerous autoimmune reactions, slow down your cellular metabolism and fat burning, and they also put a strain on your kidneys, liver, and spleen.

Detoxing is a process in which you help your body get rid of all harmful substances.

However, there are numerous misconceptions about detoxing. Sadly, many people think that they're doing their bodies a favor if they spend a week to ten days eating nothing but juice. Yikes, this isn't good. Your body can do very little to heal without solid macronutrients like protein and healthy fats. You should never deprive yourself of food unless mandated by your doctor. However, in some cases, your body might need a gentle nudge to process metabolic byproducts faster and to neutralize and expel toxins that found their way into your blood.

This is where detoxing kicks in as a useful tool to support the natural detoxing processes. Despite general belief, your body knows how to detox itself quite well. In fact, there's a whole range of mechanisms; from intestinal flora to your inner organ functioning, and even how your cardiovascular system operates, that are designed to cleanse your body.

You're not trying to physically flush your body of toxins while detoxing. You are, however, providing crucial support for your body's natural mechanisms to perform well. These mechanisms may have slowed down as a result of the toxic overwhelm that happens when you eat too many store-bought foods that contain toxic chemicals. Your body has, indeed, only been equipped to filter natural toxins. It could use more help with getting rid of the industrial ones though, as they're more persistent, heavy-duty, and harder to break down.

Juicing can help! In this chapter, you'll learn how to make cleansing beverages that empower your body to break down and eject excess toxins.

CARROT AND APPLE JUICE

These two flavors complement each other and work together amazingly. Plus, both fruits are considered to be nutrient bombs! It will take you a total of 10 minutes to prepare one glass of this cleansing potion with your juicer. However, the benefits of the juice are overwhelming. It protects your heart health, boosts your immune system, and more importantly, helps your body get rid of all the toxins and unhealthy substances that may have been piling up.

Ingredients:

The ingredients you will need for this juice include:

- Two cups of baby carrots
- Two quartered apples
- Two stalks of celery
- One piece of fresh ginger that's about a half-inch long

Directions:

First, wash all of the products and choose whether or not you wish to keep or remove the peels. After that, begin inserting the carrots, apples, and celery into the juicer and then add ginger.

This delicious juice has no more than 277 calories.

Juicing Tips:

If you wish to alter some of the ingredients, in this case, you can substitute apples or any other sweet-tasting fruit or vegetable that you like. This includes beats or pears.

Equipment and Storage

If it weren't for the delicious carrots in this juice, I'd freely approve of storing it for up to 48 hours. However, the sweetness of this particular vegetable calls for caution, so I'd advise storing it for no longer than 24 hours in your vacuum container. Aside from that, you'll need your magic juicer, a sharp knife, and a board to cut on.

APPLE, GINGER, AND LEMON JUICE CLEANSER

To truly cleanse and detoxify your body, you will greatly benefit from this sweet, yet strong-tasting juice made of apples, ginger, lemon, and cayenne pepper. Similar to the other juice recipes, this one will take approximately 15 minutes to complete.

First, wash and cut your apples, lemons and ginger. You can always keep the skins if you like. Remember to core the apples or extract the seeds if you want to avoid adding that bitter seed flavor.

Run all the ingredients through your juicer, starting with apples and finishing with ginger and cayenne.

A pinch of cayenne is all you need given how the juicing process works. I would recommend adding Cayenne to your glass once the juice is already finished.

Ingredients:

For this recipe, you will need:

- 16 ounces of carrots
- Two apples,
- Half of a medium lemon
- Half an inch chunk of ginger

Juicing Tips

Don't forget to wash the produce! In this case, peel the lemon because it could add some bitterness to the juice beet and ginger juice. If you were looking for a delicious way to detox, this neat recipe is all you need.

Equipment and Storage

Drink your juice within 24 hours. Equipment needed for this carroty delight includes your juicer, a vacuum container, a sharp knife, and a bamboo board.

BEETROOT AND GINGER JUICE

This time, you will enjoy a rich flavor that blends the aromas of parsley, beetroot, ginger, apples, and lemon into a vibrant antioxidant drink that's filled with vitamins and minerals to your taste.

Ingredients

For this juice, you'll need:

- Raw beets to taste
- One apple
- A half-inch piece of fresh ginger
- Approximately half a cup of organic parsley
- Half of a fresh lemon

Instructions:

First, wash and prep all of the ingredients and then pop them into your juicer. This amazing juice will help improve your blood flow and it will also help control blood pressure. It will give your liver a gentle nudge to continue successfully detoxifying chemicals from your body, and it will also help you increase your muscle strength.

Equipment and Storage:

Given that the ingredients in this juice are long-lasting, you can take the liberty of storing it in a vacuum container for up to 48 hours. Make sure that you have your clean juicer nearby, as well as a cutting board, knife, and an apple corer to extract seeds. You'll also need a quality peeler, should you choose to get rid of skins.

GREEN DETOX CLEANSE JUICE

This amazing juice takes no longer than 10 minutes to prepare approximately 16 ounces of the beverage.

Ingredients

You will need:

- 10 leaves of kale
- A small handful of spinach leaves
- One medium cucumber
- A couple of small apples
- One inch piece of ginger and one half of a lime

The process is simple from here on. All you need to do is wash all of your ingredients thoroughly with water.

Prepping Tips

You can soak kale, spinach, cucumber, and apples in a bowl of water for no longer than three minutes. If you're intent on getting them extra clean, you can also add a teaspoon of baking soda. I recommend doing this if you want to keep your apple and cucumber skins, which enhance the richness of nutrients that they contain. After you've washed your ingredients, you can chop the apples and the cucumber into two halves or quarters depending on how you like best. After that, you can insert them into your juicer and begin juicing away to a delicious glass of highly detoxing beverage.

Juicing Tips

I recommend coring the apples to avoid adding bitterness to the juice. I also recommend first juicing the spinach and kale and then adding ginger apples, limes, and cucumbers. While this juice should be drunk quickly after making, you can let it sit in your refrigerator for a couple of minutes and keep it there just long enough to cool down.

Equipment and Storage

Your peeler, juicer, knife, and cutting board will suffice to make this juice. Given how the ingredients in it will quickly decay, I'd recommend either drinking it right away or storing it for up to 24 hours.

MINT CUCUMBER DETOX

Ingredients:

This delicious recipe includes:

- About three liters of water
- Half a cucumber
- A couple of slices of lemons
- Up to 12 mint leaves

Instructions:

Insert your cucumber, mint, and lemon slices and juice away! Towards the end of the process, run the water through your juicer to get all of the veggie residues.

Juicing Tips:

As you can see, this detox is intended to be consumed throughout the entire day. This means that you don't have to drink an entire gallon of it for your single serving. Instead, this recipe gives you six servings of this delicious juice.

Equipment and Storage:

You'll need a peeler if you wish to get rid of lemon peels. Aside from that, you'll make good use of a bamboo cutting board, a rust-resistant knife, and as always, your juicer. You can let this refreshing beverage cool down and sit in the fridge throughout the entire day.

KALE AND LEMON JUICE

The benefits of drinking lemon water early in the morning have been widely discussed, and a consensus is that this simple ritual helps boost digestion, and more importantly, reduces appetite.

Lemon water is also found to be helpful if you are on an intermittent fasting regimen and you need to find a way to keep yourself from eating when you are fasting. This drink is also a natural detoxifier that will refresh your body and boost your immune system.

Ingredients:

- Two cups of chopped kale
- Up to two liters of water
- One to two lemons
- A couple of leaves of mint

Instructions:

The food prep for this juice is quite easy. All you need to do is soak your ingredients briefly in water or rinse them in their tepid water and then pop them all together into your juicer.

Juicing Tips:

You should drink this juice slowly throughout the day. No rush! Have a glass before, after, and in between meals.

Equipment and Storage:

You'll need your juicer, cutting board, and knife to make this detox. You can let it sit in your fridge for the entire day.

ORANGE AND CARROT DETOX

This yummy treat includes complimenting flavors that can also be combined with additional fruits per your taste.

Ingredients:

For this recipe, you will need:

- Two to three cut-up carrots
- A tablespoon of ginger
- A tablespoon of turmeric
- One tablespoon of lemon juice

Instructions:

The process from here on is simple. First, wash your ingredients thoroughly and then peel the oranges and carrots. Cut them into halves or quarters and begin making your juice. I recommend only juicing carrots and oranges while adding lemon juice, turmeric, and ginger afterward into your glass. This will prevent these precious ingredients from getting mixed up with the pulp and eventually not finding their way into your juice.

Juicing Tips:

While I do recommend trying to keep the skins, in this case, they might spoil the taste of the juice a little bit. As usual, use the skins only if you don't mind a bit of bitterness to secure extra nutrition.

Another fun way to make this juice is to press carrots and oranges separately. While this one small change can truly impact the taste or detoxifying properties of the juice, it could also be helpful since the two fruits have different consistencies. Some juicers may not mix all of the ingredients well, which is why separating them is useful.

Equipment and Storage

You need the basic juicing equipment which consists of your knife, board, and juicer. If you wish to peel carrots thoroughly, then you'll also need a peeler. I recommend drinking this juice within 24 hours.

GINGER ALE

Ginger ale has a long tradition and history, and it's popular with people from many cultures across different ages. However, I don't recommend drinking ginger ale from your local stores, as it likely doesn't have all the nutritional properties of homemade ginger ale. What's great about this recipe is that it will take you only two minutes to create over a liter of ginger ale.

Ingredients

For this recipe, you will need:

- A chunk of ginger that is approximately 10 centimeters long
- One whole lemon
- A liter of mineral water
- Two tablespoons of maple syrup

Prepping Tips

The preparation here is simple as well. Leave the skin on your ginger and cut it into small pieces. To prep your lemons, remove their ends and try keeping the skin if you don't mind a slightly bitter taste.

Instructions

Mix the ingredients inside the juicer. Add the ginger first and later insert the lemons. Enjoy watching as the juice is being made!

Juicing Tips

Add the maple syrup only once approximately half of the ingredients have been processed. Next, pour the mineral water through the juicer so that it will pick up all of the remaining ingredients. Let the bowl fill and only release the juice to the jug after a minute or two has passed. Add the remaining mineral water to the jug.

Equipment and Storage

As usual, you'll need a juicer, a bamboo board, and a knife. Feel free to savor the drink throughout the whole day while letting it sit inside your fridge.

ALLERGY-FIGHTING GREEN DETOX JUICE

Allergies are frequent companions of people who struggle with obesity and chronic diseases. Allergies are autoimmune illnesses that usually occur once one's immune system is overwhelmed by irritants and pathogens for a prolonged time. Obesity can happen as a result of damaged intestinal flora. After years of eating unhealthy foods, your intestinal flora, or rather the bacteria and beneficial fungi, and other microorganisms that protect your intestines, no longer receive the necessary nutrition to thrive and stay diverse. They begin dying off. What happens next? You get a syndrome called a leaky gut. A leaky gut is linked with immune deficiencies, hormonal imbalances, insulin resistance, and mainly autoimmune reactions. Now, why are autoimmune reactions common in this scenario? When you have a leaky gut, your intestine allows toxins, dirt, and pathogens from your food to pass into your bloodstream. That way, your immune system becomes overly active. Once this occurs for a longer period, your body's immune system begins reacting to nutrients and other substances that otherwise aren't harmful to your body. This is one of the main reasons why people develop chronic allergies nowadays.

How can juicing help? Certain foods are said to be able to quell an overactive immune system and relieve allergies by replenishing intestinal flora. This juice will take only 10 minutes to make for a single serving.

Ingredients:

This juice includes:

- Parsley
- One bunch of light leaves
- One scrubbed medium cucumber
- Two medium peeled lemons
- One cored apple
- An inch of fresh ginger root to sweeten the pot
- A teaspoon of raw honey or five drops of liquid stevia.

Directions

First, wash and chop all of your ingredients and then push them through the juicer.

Juicing Tips

Before drinking, make sure to dilute the juice with a cup of filtered water.

Equipment and Instructions

Aside from your juicer, knife, and cutting board, you'll need an apple corer. Make sure to drink your juice on the same day!

HERBAL GREEN DETOX

Are you looking for some natural sweetness that won't spike your blood sugar, but will still be a delicious treat in the middle of a hard day's work? In that case, I recommend choosing this delicious cucumber and ginger juice with spinach, parsley, and apples that will detox your body and still taste amazing.

Ingredients:

For this recipe, you will need:

- One inch of fresh ginger that's been thoroughly cleaned and scrubbed, so that you can juice the precious skin
- One medium lemon

Instructions:

The process of juicing is simple. Begin with apples, spinach, parsley, and lemon, then add ginger so that it is properly distributed across the liquid. When it comes to lemons, you also have the choice between using the skin or throwing it away if you don't want the altered flavor.

Equipment and Storage

If you're not a fan of skins, you'll need a peeler to thoroughly clean your ginger and lemon. Aside from that, you'll need your star cold-press juicer, a plain knife, bamboo board, and of course, a vacuum container if you wish to store the juice for up to 48 hours.

Boy, aren't these cleanses delicious? I bet you never thought that detoxing could be so easy and fun. Before you learn more about making juices to treat various aches and pains, there are some important things to remember about detoxing. Remember that detoxing is still supplementation. You should account for the few calories that it will bring to your diet, since only about an extra 20 cal is enough to start gaining weight long-term. Still, don't reduce your diet or apply calorie restrictions for the sake of detoxing. This isn't necessary! Make sure to eat a healthy, clean diet, while the amazing detox recipes given in this chapter do their trick.

Now, onto the next venture. While detoxing will help you clear toxins from your body, you might still struggle with one too many aches and pains. In the next chapter, you'll learn how to cope with those with the help of juicing.

7

JUICING FOR COMMON AILMENTS

W ait... Juices can help treat illnesses? If you ever had a cold in a state when you shouldn't take medication, you wouldn't doubt juice for a second! Let me tell you a story about a friend who got a terrible cold, but couldn't get medication for medically justified reasons. When your doctor checks your throat and says 'ouch', you know you're not doing well. However, given the circumstances of her health condition, she got a recommendation to try and recover via diet and hydration, and gave it a couple more days before using medication. 'Diet?,' she thought to herself, 'I can barely swallow a sip of water, let alone a salad.' For someone who hasn't yet gotten used to juicing, it was a true refreshment (pun intended) to realize that she could take a bunch of fruits and veggies all at once, and have an entire pot of veggies within a single glass. Determined to try and follow through with her doctor's advice, my friend took one big glass of juice with pulp in the afternoon, and one in the evening.

Later that night, she noticed that she was sweating a bit more and her fever had gone down. She was able to breathe comfortably again, and her throat was no longer sore. She was a whole new person in the morning. The cold had cleared entirely, and my friend was, by all accounts, completely healthy. While we both remain with full faith in modern medicine, I couldn't help but wonder if over-medicating–which is something we do if we hop right onto the pharmacy wagon without even trying to boost the immune system, actually prevents the body from healing. If you look at what happens to your body when you're sick, you'll realize just how essential nutrition is to recover.

Our bodies rely on the immune system to fight off illnesses, and there are also dozens of physiological healing processes in store for the majority of diseases that you might get. Your body has already designed all sorts of defense strategies from pathogens, but are those mechanisms operating correctly and as nature intended? Remember, your immune system is well capable of battling illnesses, but it depends on nutrients to work properly. If we're being honest, most people nowadays don't eat as many fruits and veggies as needed for the body to be able to heal naturally.

This is where juicing kicks in as a nutrient bomb that supports your digestion, gut health, hormonal balance, and immune system. The nutrients that you obtain from the juice are fuel for the body to heal. Aside from supporting the body's natural healing processes, juicing can help with the following ailments:

- **Chronic pain.** There are many types of chronic pain that are either directly or indirectly associated with nutrient deficiencies. You can suffer from gas, bloating, and cramps as a result of hormonal imbalance and indigestion, which are associated with nutrition. Headaches and migraines, for example, are often said to alleviate after a person makes beneficial changes to their diet. Muscle and joint pain are also said to alleviate with the increase in the right nutrients, like magnesium, iron, calcium, Vitamin B complex, omega 3 fatty acids, and others. The mechanisms that govern what we perceive as pain are far too complex to discuss in this book. However, nutrition was found to affect the reduction of hormones and neurotransmitters that create the sensation of pain, and to enhance those body and brain chemicals that make us feel well-rested, relaxed, and rejuvenated.

- **Allergies and irritation.** At the very least, the juice helps get an abundant dose of nutrients that alleviate symptoms of allergies. However, juicing can truly help reduce and recover from allergies in the long term by healing your gut microbiota. Gut health is considered a significant contributor to preventing allergies, as healthy intestinal microorganisms prevent irritants from entering your blood, and activate your immune system.

- **Disease prevention and alleviation.** Most of the time, you hear about life-threatening illnesses only being discovered in their advanced stages. By the time the disease is discovered, it is so advanced that it begins to cause symptoms and various pains that severely impact one's quality of life. Before diseases become advanced, they can manifest themselves in the form of localized pain, joint pain, muscle cramps across different parts of the body, and many other symptoms. It's important to note that these alarming symptoms mean that you should check your health more thoroughly. However, any concerning symptoms are also to be treated so as to be able to proceed with a fulfilling life. A lot of the time, the medication given to treat symptoms of illness doesn't fully work. For example, migraines can occur as a symptom and side-effect of various illnesses. Taking medications for them long-term often isn't recommended to avoid developing resistance or addiction. In cases like these, nutrients can help manage concerning symptoms. A similar case goes for irritations and skin diseases that have quite limited options to treat with medication and ointments. There's a long list of illnesses that, in order to fully recover, require that a person thoroughly changes their diet. Vitamin and mineral deficiency is considered to be a significant contributor to developing chronic illness, meaning that a rich dose of nutrients helps maintain any health improvement achieved with medication.

With this in mind, below are the top juice recipes that help cope with illness.

APPLE LEMON GINGER JUICE

This amazing juice features only 155 calories within a 12-ounce serving. It takes no more than 15 minutes to prepare. It helps boost your health, support your immune system, promote weight loss, and overall helps you feel more energized.

Ingredients:

- Two and one-quarter of red apples
- Half of a medium lemon
- A half an inch piece of ginger
- A pinch of ground cayenne

Prepping Tips

To prepare this juice, start by washing the produce and making sure that you have enough of the required ingredients. Make sure to remove the seeds if you don't want your juice to taste more bitter. However, if you don't mind changes in the taste, you can leave the skins and juice all of the ingredients.

Instructions

Add the apples first, and follow up with lemon and ginger. Add a pinch of cayenne to the glass.

Juicing Tips

As always, proper washing is necessary, especially if you want to leave the skins on and benefit from their amazing nutrients. While this is recommended, be weary of germs and bacteria that are easily transferred. Lemon juice is a natural alkalizer that helps your metabolism and cancer prevention.

Equipment and Storage

While I recommend drinking this juice within a day, you may extend its lifespan by adding more ginger and lemons, given that you store the juice in your favorite vacuum container. Use the best juicer, knife, and cutting board you have!

GREEN DETOX JUICE

What, yet another green detox? You can never have too many beverages made to replenish your body! The reason why there are so many detox juices is that there's a variety of ingredients that contribute to detoxing, and many of them contain potent antioxidants that serve different purposes.

This juice, for example, features spinach, mint, mango, parsley, and oranges, with only a pinch of salt to season the mix.

Ingredients:

- One and a quarter cups of spinach
- A cup of orange juice

- A quarter cup of mint leaves
- A quarter cup of mint and parsley
- One and a quarter cups of mango

Prepping Tips

To prepare the ingredients, soak the spinach and parsley briefly in water and soak for only a minute or two.

You can also briefly rinse them if that's what you prefer.

Instructions

Run your spinach, mango, celery, mint, and parsley through the juicer and add a cup of orange juice and salt to your glass.

Juicing Tips

You can also puree ingredients if you don't want to run your mango through the juicer. Mango is a sort of fatty fruit that isn't known for juicing successfully. So, you want to avoid running it through the press, which could send most of it to the pulp instead of into the glass.

Another useful tip is to add a cup of a couple of fresh mint leaves to the glass of anti-inflammatory juice.

If you're coping with frequent inflammations, then this juice can be a great help.

Equipment and Storage

You'll need a sharp knife and a cutting board to prep your ingredients, as well as a bowl to soak in if needed. If you wish to store your juice for up to 48 hours, grab your best vacuum container!

PINEAPPLE COUGH SOLUTION

Need help with your persistent cough? This amazing recipe helps you soothe throat irritation comfortably while enjoying a delicious treat.

Ingredients

The main ingredients include:

- Four stalks of celery
- Half a cucumber
- One cup of diced pineapple
- Half of a green apple
- A cup of spinach,
- A one-inch chunk of ginger
- One lemon.

Prepping Tips

First, rinse your celery, cucumber, apple, and spinach by running them quickly through water and then peel the lemon. You can also leave the peel on the ginger.

Directions

Run all the ingredients through your juicer and alternate between celery, cucumber, pineapple, and the rest of the ingredients. Add ginger towards the end of the process.

Juicing Tips

If you don't want your juice to be overly spicy, feel free to reduce the amount of ginger.

Equipment and Storage

Aside from your favorite container in which you'll store the solution for up to 48 hours, you'll need a pineapple corer, a sharp knife, a bamboo cutting board, and of course, your cold-press juicer.

BLOOD CLEANSING JUICE

Now you must be wondering, what are the things that you should cleanse your blood from? Well, as it turns out, our blood contains toxins, irritants, as well as fats and triglycerides. Ingredients like green apples, parsley, lime, celery, ginger, and lemons are all incredibly potent and will have a deeply detoxifying effect on your body.

Ingredients

For this amazing juice, you will need:

- Five kale leaves
- One green apple
- One lime
- One lemon
- A bunch of celery

Also, bring one inch of fresh ginger to the table.

Prepping Tips

Start making your juice by properly cleaning and prepping the ingredients. Wash celery and then rinse your green apple, lemon, lime, parsley, and kale. If you wish to leave the peels on the lemon and lime, you can briefly soak them in water with a little bit of baking soda.

Instructions

As always, you can add ingredients to your juicer by rotating the softer ones with the harder ones. This will ensure that all of the ingredients are being equally processed!

Juicing Tips

You can either alternate your ingredients in the juicer or juice them one after another. However, I would always recommend alternating the ingredients to avoid the harder produce making it difficult to juice the softer ones or clogging the juicer.

Equipment and Storage

Drink your juice during the first 48 hours of making it. Store in the refrigerator while in your favorite container. You need basic equipment for cutting and juicing.

ROOT JUICE

If one of your goals, in addition to weight loss, is to replenish and rejuvenate your body, then you have to try this amazing group to juice. The secret of this juice is that it conveniently consists of root plants or root vegetables. The veggies in this juice include carrots while the fruit part of it consists of blood oranges. You will also use some spicy turmeric and ginger. This juice will contain no gluten, no grains or other allergens, and it will also be potent with nutrients that are otherwise found in these amazing plants.

Ingredients

You will need:

- One medium chopped and peeled beet
- Three medium sides of chopped and scraped carrots
- One seedless blood orange
- A two-inch piece of turmeric root and a one-inch piece of fresh ginger
- A pinch of black pepper and cayenne pepper
- Half of a lemon

Prepping Tips

Make sure to remove the skins and take out the seeds.

Directions

The juicing process, once again, couldn't be simpler. All you need to do is run the ingredients through the juicer. Given that the entire juice is a mix of root plants, I wouldn't necessarily recommend mixing them all. In this case, it might be recommended to choose one ingredient after another to keep the consistency and potency of each ingredient.

Juicing Tips

I recommend adding cayenne pepper and black pepper directly into the glass instead of adding them to the juicer. Stirring the spices and mixing the ingredients so that the whole of the juice is equal consistency.

Equipment and Storage

Keep your juice refrigerated in a vacuum container for no longer than 48 hours. Prepare your peeler, corer, board, knife, and juicer for making this recipe.

PAIN RELIEVING JUICE

This juice doesn't only help relieve inflammation. It also helps relieve pain. If you're coping with any type of chronic pain, this delicious juice can be a great help. This recipe has been said to help manage arthritis pain, as well as help your body recover from chronic illnesses like heart disease and cancer. The abundant antioxidants found in this beverage will help boost your immune system as well relieve any chronic nausea.

Also, the recipe is safe for anyone who copes with chronic allergies and are looking for a safe, long-term solution to turn to amid allergy breakouts.

Ingredients

For this juice, you will need:

- One cup of sliced or diced pineapple
- One large carrot
- Two medium stalks of celery
- One and a half inches or two teaspoons of turmeric
- A quarter teaspoon of black pepper
- A quarter cup of pomegranate juice
- A half cup of water
- A bit of ice
- A one-inch piece of ginger

Instructions

First, blend all of the ingredients in your juicer and start juicing as you normally would. Start with the pineapple, and then insert your carrots, celery, turmeric, and pomegranate, and run some water through the juicer to rinse any residue. Finally, once you've stirred all of the ingredients together, add black pepper.

Juicing Tips

I recommend adding the pulp to your juicer because it will further boost the nutrient benefits of this drink.

Equipment and Storage

Your juice should be refrigerated if you allow it to sit for up to a day–in a vacuum container. As always, have your juicer, board, peeler, and knife ready.

THE LIVER DETOX JUICE

Let's detox your liver with this beautiful blush juice that's free of gluten and features a dazzling cilantro beet flavor!

Ingredients

The ingredients that you'll need include:

- One medium size beat
- Six stalks of celery
- One cup of fresh cilantro
- One half of a lemon
- One-inch piece ginger

Instructions

As per previous instructions, insert all of the ingredients into the juicer and let the magic take place. You can keep the skins on your beets and ginger as long as you have washed and sanitized them properly.

Equipment and Storage

This juice is more beneficial when consumed immediately. So, instead of letting it sit in the fridge, get to drinking right away. You don't need any specific tools, except for your standard juicing equipment.

Juicing Tips

I recommend making this juice first thing in the morning and drinking it on an empty stomach.

PINEAPPLE COUGH SUPPRESSANT

If you were looking for an organic way to treat coughs, look no further. This pineapple syrup is outstanding! It will only take you five minutes to make approximately a half liter of this juice. It will help you with symptoms of a cold, while the delicious pineapple flavor will be a far more pleasant alternative to your chemically-tasting medications.

Ingredients

- Half of a cored apple
- Sliced lemon
- Two table teaspoons of manuka honey

Prepping Tips

To prep, cut your pineapple to the top and the bottom. You can use the corner to cut into the fruit and extract around half of it. If you wish to use the whole pineapple, you can make a double dose of the juice or you can also prep the entire pineapple and simply freeze the remainder of the fruit.

Cut the fruit either into long stripes or concentric circles, like you otherwise would when using a corer.

Instructions

Next, chop the pineapple and prepare the lemon. Remove the top and the bottom from the fruit and slice it. Begin juicing the pineapple and gradually run it through the juicer. The core should be juiced with a couple of pieces at a time. Finish off with slices of lemon.

Heat one medium saucepan to body temperature and test the heat with the tip of your finger.

Juicing Tips

Pour the juice inside and let it steam but not boil, since boiling will, or could ruin all the nutritional potency. Then drink the juice immediately.

Equipment and Storage

It's best to use the cough solution immediately after making it. If you choose to make larger quantities, be mindful to only heat at the lightest temperatures and to never let the juice boil. Aside from a vacuum container to store the juice, you'll also need a saucepan, knife, corer, and a cutting board.

ALLERGY-RELIEVING CILANTRO JUICE

This juice is another great solution for anyone needing to reduce or alleviate their allergies.

Ingredients

- Two tablespoons of aloe vera gel
- One cup of raw chopped cabbage
- Half a cup of cilantro

Instructions

First, juice your cabbage and cilantro together.

If you wish for a milder taste, you can run a cup of water through the juicer. Lastly, add the aloe vera gel and stir it into the juice.

Juicing Tips

Feel free to add a tablespoon of lemon juice if you wish to enhance the flavor!

Equipment and Storage

Drink your juice either immediately upon making it or within the first 24 hours. If you're storing your juice, do so in a vacuum container. You don't need any special equipment aside from your standard juicing tools.

TANGY GREENS AND APPLE JUICE

Who says that all the healthiest juices must also be bitter and poor-tasting? In this recipe, you'll learn to make delicious apple and ginger juice that will be as healing as it is yummy.

Ingredients

For this gingery green delight, you'll need:

- Two to three whole green apples
- One cucumber
- One whole lemon
- An inch-long piece of fresh ginger
- A handful of baby spinach leaves

Prepping Tips

You can soak your apples and lemon briefly if you wish to keep the skins. If not, rinse them with water and peel them. Rinse your baby spinach as well.

Core the apples and cut them into small pieces, along with the lemon.

Instructions

Begin by juicing the apples and the lemon. Add the baby spinach and ginger about halfway through the process.

Juicing Tips

If you wish for the drink to taste spicy, add more ginger. If you want to increase the sweetness, add a bit more apple.

Wow, just look at how many juices you can now make! In this chapter, you learned to make juices that will help you relieve pain, allergy, cough, and much more. Juicing can help you recover from colds as well, just make sure to consult your doctor before making any medication decisions.

You've almost made it to the end of your juicing manual. The previous chapters have taught you what to do for successful juicing in grave detail. From using your juicer to combining foods, you now know how to manage your product like a genuine professional. Juicing is supposed to be light, easy, and more importantly, effective, for years to come. If you start experiencing health problems, or you don't see the benefits you were hoping to see, you might not feel completely happy. This is why the next chapter will be all about avoiding key mistakes with juicing.

8

THE JUICING JEOPARDIES

Do you want to be successful with juicing? If so, the process isn't as simple as "beating the food to a pulp" and gulping the juice down all at once. People who do so face all the risks associated with careless juicing, like weight gain and increased blood sugar. As you have learned by now, the main benefits of juicing revolve around the impact of nutrients on your body's physiological processes and cellular health. However, such crucial benefits don't come easily. You need to be careful about how you drink your juice, what foods you use, and how you store your juice if you want to get the most out of the process.

More importantly, you should be mindful of the following juicing mistakes that you should avoid making (Are You Making These 8 Common Juicing Mistakes?, n.d.):

MISTAKE #1: NOT DRINKING YOUR JUICE WHILE FRESH

Your juice is the most potent right after making it. As the minutes go by, so do many beneficial nutrients in your juice, as they begin to deteriorate. Keep in mind that an average juice, made from multiple foods, contains dozens of nutrients that we can confidently say benefit your health, plus many that are rare. Throughout this book, you learned about foods that contain rare nutrients, like ginger, pineapple, carrots, and leafy greens. It's difficult to obtain the needed amount of these nutrients through daily eating, and for several reasons listed below.

Nutrients decay quickly. Your vitamins, minerals, and phyto proteins can live a long, healthy life inside a fruit. There, they're packed inside all sorts of membranes made from pulp substances, and they're organized in tissue units that are similar to how tissues are organized and grouped inside a human body. When you put foods through a juicer, you're removing all of the natural structure that holds the nutrients together. The nutrients, when exposed to air, start to die off within minutes.

Nutrients oxidize. Raw nutrients found in juice start reacting with oxygen within minutes. This reaction is similar to what happens to fruit immediately after peeling and cutting. You've probably noticed that a fruit salad, for example, no longer tastes good even 10-15 minutes after eating. Oxidation kills off many of your nutrients, and it also creates harmful free radicals, which are associated with cellular damage and many life-threatening illnesses.

Temperature and germs harm your nutrients. Room temperature is a fertile ground for all sorts of germs, which is why we're often warned against leaving food outside the fridge for longer than a couple of minutes. Now, it would be an exaggeration to say that you can get a serious infection. However, bacteria and fungi can feed off of your juice and begin to ferment it, which slightly affects nutrient composition. This isn't a problem if you're drinking juice only occasionally. However, if you're juicing for months at a time, and you're taking multiple servings of juice each day, the slight increases in sugar can amount to significant ones over time.

MISTAKE #2: YOUR JUICE HAS TOO MUCH-PROCESSED SUGAR

Yes, it is possible to unknowingly add processed sugar to your juice. This can happen in the following circumstances.

You're adding store-bought condiments. You might feel tempted to add condiments to enhance the flavor of your juice. You might be particularly tempted to do so if you drink juices solely based on nutrition labels and without paying attention to how different flavors will work together. However, adding store-bought ingredients to your juice could be a grave mistake. The condiments and sweeteners could easily contain a lot more sugar than you should be taking. Or, they might contain corn starch, which gets broken down into sugar when digested. Keep this in mind and make sure that your juice tastes nice before adding anything to it.

You're using too much fruit. You can easily spike the amount of sugar in your juice by adding one too many fruits. This is particularly possible if you muster the strength to give up snacks and candy, so juice becomes your only source of sugar. Be mindful of your fruit's nutrient composition, and calculate how much sugar goes into your juice. That way, you'll avoid that awkward realization that you've been kicking your blood sugar out of balance and gaining weight, all while thinking that you've found a life-transforming route.

You're using pre-packaged goods. Similar to adding condiments to your juice, you might feel tempted to buy frozen, pre-packaged, canned, or otherwise pre-made fruits and vegetables. After all, food prep can take a long time, and having food that you can simply pour out of a bag or a can right into your juicer is tempting. Avoid doing this unless you're extremely skillful at monitoring and calculating nutrient intake. Stores don't separate those foods that have been packaged healthfully from those that have chemicals added to enhance flavor and shelf life. It is a piece of information that you're going to have to discover on your own. If you're shopping for frozen or packaged produce, check nutrition labels to see if any food dyes, aromas, or sweeteners were added to the mix.

MISTAKE #3: IT'S NOT COLD-PRESSED

As you learned in the first two chapters of this book, cold-pressed juicers yield a lot better quality of juice compared to other juicers. One of the reasons why you might be cautious against cold-pressed juicers is the amount of time and effort needed to make juice. It is true that cold-pressed juicers take longer to make juice, and that you need to be more mindful of how you're inserting produce, how much produce you're adding to the juicer, and how thoroughly you clean your juice.

However, cold-pressed juicers enhance the flavor and quality of your juice in multiple ways:

- They eliminate air. The lack of air inside the press and the auger means two important things. First, your juice doesn't start to oxidize early into the juicing process. Oxidation kills off the nutrients and mellows the juice flavor, and this is why juices made with the cold-press technology taste a lot better. Second, the lack of air while juicing also means that there are fewer bacteria and other pathogens in your juice. This is particularly important if you're drinking a lot of homemade juice every day.
- More juice. Cold-press juicers are more potent when it comes to extracting liquid from food. They don't strictly rely on chopping the food using the blade, but instead they grind your food to get the most juice out of it. This is the main reason why an average person is now able to juice root plants and other harder produce with the same success as they do soft fruits and citruses. Cold-pressed juicers produce significantly more juice compared to

alternatives, and it's a shame to miss out on the benefits.

- Easier operating. Cold-pressed juicers can process larger quantities and more varieties when it comes to production. You don't have to limit juicing to only one or two ingredients. Instead, if you're only making one or two servings, you can mix the foods, and the juicer will process them all quite evenly. Plus, cold-pressed juicers are less wasteful. They press the produce powerfully and leave you with almost dehydrated pulp that you can later either use or toss, per your taste.

MISTAKE #4: YOU'RE NOT DRINKING JUICE ON AN EMPTY STOMACH

Drinking juice on an empty stomach is essential to feel comfortable and to absorb as many nutrients as possible. If you don't drink your green juice on an empty stomach, you might even get heartburn. Drinking fresh juice on an empty stomach helps replenish your intestinal flora, and begins to heal it so that you can start to regain hormonal balance. If you recall, in one of the earlier chapters, we talked about leaky gut. With a leaky gut, you have a reduced capacity to absorb nutrients. Contrary to what people think, nutrients aren't absorbed straight from the stomach and into the blood and tissues. A good portion of them are, but an even bigger portion serves as food to the gut biota, which is a process in which nutrients are synthesized into many enzymes and hormones needed for your body to function properly. So, you might visualize that vitamins go into your stomach and straight into your blood and cells, but that's not the case. Without a well-functioning microbiota, it's a lot harder for the body to produce serotonin, dopamine, melatonin, endorphins, testosterone, progesterone, estrogen, and other hormones that affect well-being. One of the biggest benefits of drinking juice on an empty stomach, as recommended some 20 minutes before a meal, is to feed and grow the helpful colonies of microorganisms in your gut. When you combine the juice with meals or drink it on a full stomach, the enzymes used to digest food can destroy many of the nutrients. When you drink juice after your body has fasted for some hours during the night, the nutrients from the juice are the first thing that enters your stomach. They go straight into your intestines and get absorbed quickly, thus "fertilizing" or feeding microbiota.

Now, it is possible that certain fruits or vegetables don't feel good on an empty stomach, and can cause heartburn. This is highly individual, and if it happens, simply look for a more suitable morning juice recipe. For example, citruses are known to cause heartburn in some people, as can apples. Raw kale, as nourishing as it is, can give some people gas. The same goes for cabbage. However, this doesn't mean that you should exclude those foods completely. You can reduce the amounts, add a bit of honey to your juice, or simply swap them for equally nourishing alternatives.

MISTAKE #5: NOT PREPARING THE INGREDIENTS PRIOR TO JUICING

No matter what the manufacturer's instructions say, avoid popping whole apples, cucumbers, lemons, and other fruits into your juicer. This isn't only a matter of juicer capacity. Indeed, some of these neat machines will chew up anything that you throw in, but what will be the quality of the juice? Even if you don't damage your press, it's questionable if you'll get the maximum juice without proper food prep.

Washing your produce ensures that no toxins and dirt end up in your juice. This makes your juice safer to consume each day, which is even more important if you're serving juice to your friends, family, or children.

Peeling and cutting the ends of the foods, as well as the parts of them that are rotten, ensures that your juice consists only of clean, healthy nutrients. It also improves the color and texture of your juice.

MISTAKE #6: USING THE WRONG JUICER

As you learned at the beginning of this book, there are many types of juicers. While I recommend a cold-press juicer, there are dozens of varieties of those as well. Juicers differentiate by whether they're vertical or horizontal, their gears and capacities, jug, press, auger sizes, and many other features. Now, when it comes to technology, there's a general notion that you should buy as potent an apparatus as needed for the intended purpose. If you purchase a smaller juicer, with less engine power, it will work for you if you're making a glass or two of juice per day. However, if you live with more people, and plan on making a larger number of servings each day, you'll need a more powerful juicer.

MISTAKE #7: TOSSING ALL THE LEFTOVERS FROM THE FRIDGE INTO YOUR JUICE

People choosing to run completely random fruits and vegetables through their juicer are one of the bigger reasons behind failure with juicing. All of your choices should be thought-through, planned, and strategically used to secure the biggest health benefits.

MISTAKE #8: TOO MANY FRUITS AND FAR LESS VEGGIES

As you might have seen from the earlier recipes, juices can sport anywhere between 50 to 250 calories, and even more. Too much fruit in your juice can amount to unhealthy amounts of sugar and excess calories taken during the day. Granted, any juice is still a better alternative to fast food and processed sugars. However, the use of too much fruit without attention to nutritive values is largely behind some of the most common juice misconceptions and can be attributed to so many dietitians and physicians being weary of juicing and refusing to recommend it to their patients.

Remember, the whole point of juicing is to take as many raw nutrients as possible, with as little sugar as possible. To ensure that you are, study the nutrient values of the foods you're juicing. Calculate the amount of sugar and carbs, net calories, and nutrients that they contain. Keep in mind the maximum amount of sugar that you should be taking each day when making your juice, and you'll avoid going overboard.

MISTAKE #9: PICKING RECIPES AS PER TASTE VERSUS HEALTH BENEFITS

Do you know what happens when you take more nutrients than your body can absorb? They're merely filtered through your liver and kidneys. When you're choosing which juice to make solely based on its taste, you're missing the whole point of juicing, which is to address your specific health concerns and needs. Instead, start by listing your health problems and nutrition goals. Then, do some digging and list all of the foods that benefit your condition and are a better alternative to the foods you commonly use. Create a plan, or rather a schedule, of which juice you'll be making, and how often you'll drink the beverage to achieve your health goals.

That way, the health benefits will snowball over time, and you'll start to feel an improvement across the board. You'll start to feel more energized, you'll have fewer chronic aches and pains, and you'll prevent many life-threatening illnesses.

Now, you may come across a common dilemma—should you drink juices that you don't personally like because of their health benefits? The answer to that question depends on how important these benefits are for you, and just how much you dislike certain foods.

Everyone has some likes and dislikes when it comes to food, but you shouldn't force yourself to drink juices that make you feel uncomfortable or nauseous. You should feel nice and enjoy your juices, so if there are sacrifices that you choose to make, the benefits should justify that.

MISTAKE #10: YOU'RE JUICING THE WRONG WAY

As it turns out, there are many potential "wrong ways" to juice, and they include:

- Using the wrong juices. Ignoring your health and nutrition needs and drinking juices because of their popularity and online recommendations is, indeed, the wrong way to juice. Instead, aim to highly personalize your juicing habit so that it directly addresses your specific needs and concerns. Make your juicing strategic and targeted instead of random, sporadic, and spontaneous.
- Neglecting your juicer cleanliness. Avoid washing your juicer parts in a dishwasher because this isn't likely to clean it all the way through. Instead, you should be washing your juicer manually after each use.

- Following an unhealthy diet. Juicing won't help if you otherwise don't make an effort to make your nutrition and lifestyle healthier. Make sure to instill the right exercise and eating changes to benefit more from juicing.
- Eating toxic produce. Given just how many fruits and vegetables you'll be taking with juicing, your product must be healthy, whole, and clean. You should try to find those suppliers whose produce is organic and hasn't been treated with harsh chemicals and pesticides.
- Drinking your juice too quickly. You shouldn't just pour the precious juice down your throat. That's not the way to absorb the most nutrition! Instead, you should take your time and drink your juice for at least 10 to 15 minutes. You should swirl the liquid in your mouth and chew any pulp that you might come across. That way, small amounts of nutrients will gradually reach your stomach, and they'll be absorbed a lot better.

Avoid making these mistakes, and you'll find plenty of success with juicing! Now that you're approaching the very end of this easy juicing manual, let's summarize this chapter by emphasizing the basic postulates of successful juicing.

Supplementation, Not Diet

Juicing is not a fad diet. It is not intended to replace meals, nor am I recommending you spend days eating nothing but juice. Doing such drastic things might complicate your health. The lack of calories, proteins, and fat in your diet could lead to cardiovascular problems and muscle loss. Be particularly weary of combining diets with high-intensity exercise. Many people think that they'll speed up fat loss if they reduce calorie intake to close to nothing, and then work out intensely for a period of time. Doing so, and particularly relying on the juice to compensate for the lack of food, could be detrimental to your health. In the absence of protein and fats, your body might actually start to break down muscle tissue just to sustain itself. You also might experience fatigue, and even get sick from not eating. While your juice's nutritive values should be accounted into the total calorie intake, the said intake should still settle for your body's everyday needs.

Instead of relying on the juice to lose weight, use juice in such ways as to support your metabolism. Ensure that you're getting the fruits and veggies that you otherwise don't get from food, and concentrate on those foods that have been found to contain rare, but valuable nutrients.

Food Choice, Not Quantity

Juicing isn't about the amount of fruit and vegetables that you eat. You could, arguably, drink almost two liters of juice daily, but this wouldn't be healthy. To your body, drinking the food is the same as eating it. You are, technically, eating the food that you've run through the juicer. Instead of focusing on the quantity of juice that you drink each day, focus on its quality. Think more about what your body's unique needs are, and what foods from the recommended list can benefit you the most. Focusing on the selection rather than the quantity of the food you'll eat ensures that daily juicing fulfills its intended purpose.

Purpose, Not Ritual

On the topic of purpose, consider juicing to be a means to an end. You are juicing because you're trying to achieve a certain result. You might be enjoying taking photos of your juicing process and posting them online, but doing so doesn't guarantee results. Many people shift focus from purposeful acting to ritualistic making and drinking juice which isn't good. Juicing by habit, without much thought put into the foods you're juicing, frequency, and more importantly, tracking results, reduces the chance of seeing the desired outcome. Relish in your newfound morning ritual, by all means. However, stay on top of your mission and goals that you're trying to achieve. Always overview the foods you're juicing, and their nutritive values, and write down and track the changes that you're noticing. This is the only way to tell if you're juicing correctly!

Preference, Not Taste

Now, onto the matter of taste when it comes to juicing. You, like most people I know, aren't likely a passionate fan of cooked vegetables and fruits. Still, that doesn't mean that some juices won't taste better than others. Some of your juices will taste so good that you'll start wanting to make only a handful of recipes. This isn't good either. Don't limit your juice to a couple of recipes that you'll be rotating weekly. Instead, explore different foods and ingredients. If you find a specific juice that caters to your ailment but you don't like the taste, then make adjustments! Find alternatives for the ingredient that you don't like, and you'll soon find yourself wishing to try different recipes every single day.

Wow, what a job you have done! You began by learning what juicers are in the first place, and here you are now, understanding the juicing process inside-out. As we approach the end of your brief juicing class, it would be worthwhile to reflect on the essential aspects of juicing.

Juicing may be an entirely new routine, but it will successfully replace all of the harmful habits that you've held onto for so long. It might take a couple of weeks to spot the first results, but the energy and positive mood gained from increased nutrient intake will kick in pretty quickly. No more waiting! It's time to make your grocery list, and head out to buy your most preferred fruits, veggies, and herbs. Good luck!

CONCLUSION

What amazing work you did! It takes curiosity and patience to learn about an entirely new practice and commit to making lifestyle changes. You have the devotion and strength needed to succeed with juicing, so why delay?

This book was written with an average person in mind. Despite the numerous proven benefits of juicing, it's still a fact that changing your routine and introducing novelties is difficult. As you've learned, getting a quality juicer doesn't have to be that hard. Although I recommend getting a cold press juicer, you'll do well with any machine that matches your juicing needs. In this book, you'll learn that you can choose between centrifugal, masticating, and manual juicers. While you can juice all the produce recommended in this book with any of the methods, masticating juicers ensure the best juice quality. You learned that each juicing method and each machine's features come with different benefits and drawbacks. Centrifugal and manual juicers might be cheaper and work faster, but they create a ton of waste. It is a pity for nearly half of the nutrients in your food to go to waste, isn't it? However, these juicers are a good option if you prefer foods that are watery and can be squeezed well regardless of the technology. However, if you wish to juice more frequently, and you want your juice to have a rich flavor, you're better off with a masticating juicer. A masticating juicer applies pressure and grinds your food rather than cutting it. That way, more nutrients and fiber is preserved, and you get to choose whether or not you wish to keep the pulp or discard it. Furthermore, masticating juicers are great for hard produce. As you learned, beats, broccoli, apples, and others need quite a potent juicer to extract the most beneficial ingredients. Now, it's up to you to decide which juicer you want.

After learning how juicers work, you learned about the best foods that you can use for juicing. You likely learned that the recommended fruits and veggies are easily found in any store and that you don't have to spend a ton of money on them. You also learned that you can use some of the more common herbs from your pantry to not only enhance the juice flavor, but also to introduce numerous beneficial nutrients. Isn't that amazing?

More importantly, you were given clear, concise, and practical juicing instructions. The last few chapters of this book showed you which recipes to use for different intents and purposes. You can successfully juice for weight loss given that you control the amount of sugar and carbs. You can also successfully use juicing to detox your body by choosing foods that contain high levels of antioxidants, plus vitamins and minerals that support cellular metabolism. Improved cellular metabolism helps your cells break down nutrients and use them to build their elements, multiply, and build healthy tissues. Furthermore, the detoxifying effects of juice support your inner organs to process metabolic byproducts and then eject them from your body. Finally, you can use the juice to support recovery from painful and distressing conditions. Given that you refrain from making vital juicing mistakes, you'll reap all the benefits without facing many shortcomings.

On the topic of mistakes, you learned what the basic principles of successful juicing are, and what you should avoid doing at all costs. You learned that you should never drink your juice as an addition to your meal, but instead take your juice on an empty stomach or in between meals. Doing so will ensure that you don't get heartburn or gas. Plus, drinking juice on an empty stomach ensures the best nutrient absorption. Moreover, you learned that you should be mindful of why you need the foods chosen for juicing. While juice should taste good, the taste shouldn't be the main criteria of choice. You should focus more on the nutritional value of your fruits and veggies, and work around the taste in order to give your body the nutrition it needs.

Aside from that, it's crucial to drink your juice fresh. While it is true that your juice can last for up to 72 days and still maintain its nutrients, that can't be said for the majority of recipes. Your juice is the healthiest right after making it! You also learned that in order to protect your health and maximize the nutritional benefits of juicing, you should keep the sugar levels to a bare minimum. In this book, this is done with recipes that were carefully designed for tasty juice with only a little bit of sugar. In that regard, avoid making the pivotal mistake of using too much fruit when making juice. Your ingredients should be carefully planned and chosen for the nutrients to target your intended purpose for juicing.

In this book, you also learned that proper food preparation is essential for your juice's success. After all, cleaning and cutting fruits ensures that your juicer gets the most liquid out of them, with as little waste as possible.

You also learned that the quality of your juice doesn't only reside with your food choice. Your juicer plays an even bigger role. Choosing a cold-press juicer might be a costlier option, but it would guarantee that your juice is nutrient-dense and delicious. Cold press juicers don't produce heat when operating, so they preserve the maximum nutrients from your ingredients. Moreover, they block the air from entering the press and prevent germs from inhabiting your juice. Cold-press juicers also protect your juice from oxidizing. When nutrients react with oxygen, they decay and create harmful by-products, whose presence defeats the whole purpose of juicing.

Remember to take a strategic, planned-out approach to juice, and you won't regret it! Always think about nutritional values and how well the selected foods contribute to your pre-set health or weight goal.

Now, it's time to start juicing! I wish you the utmost luck and send all the positive energy and intentions for your journey! Have you found this book useful? If you did, don't forget to leave an honest review so that other readers know how you benefited from the reading.

REFERENCES

Are You Making These 8 Common Juicing Mistakes? (n.d.). Hungry for Change. Retrieved October 31, 2022, from https://www.hungryfor change.tv/article/are-you-making-these-common-8-juicing-mistakes

Brown, M. J. (2019, October 4). *Juicing: Good or Bad?* Healthline; Healthline Media. https://www.healthline.com/nutrition/juicing-good-or-bad#juicing-for-nutrients

Cross, J. (n.d.). *Produce Prep.* Joe Cross. https://www.rebootwithjoe. com/juicing/produce-prep/

Goodnature. (2020, February 25). *11 Creative Ways to Use Leftover Juice Pulp.* Goodnature. https://www.goodnature.com/blog/11-creative-ways-to-use-leftover-juice-pulp/

Juicing Herbs. (n.d.). AH Juice. Retrieved October 31, 2022, from http:// ahjuice.com/juicing-herbs-2/

Link, R. (2019, July 4). *The 12 Best Vegetables to Juice.* Healthline. https:// www.healthline.com/nutrition/best-vegetables-to-juice

Mather, K. (2014, October 1). *10 Reasons Why Juicing Can Improve Your Life.* The Body Toolkit. https://www.thebodytoolkit.com/blog-arti cle/10-reasons-why-juicing-can-improve-your-life

Panoff, L. (2020, June 5). *How to Wash Fruits and Vegetables: A Complete Guide.* Healthline. https://www.healthline.com/nutrition/washing-vegetables#why-wash-them

University, C., & University, S. (n.d.). *How to Choose a Juicer.* Treehug-ger. https://www.treehugger.com/how-to-choose-a-juicer-or-do-you-need-a-blender-4860205

Wells, N. (2019, May 29). *Top 10 Best Fruits for Juicing & How to Prepare Them (with Pictures).* House Grail. https://housegrail.com/which-fruits-are-best-for-juicing/

www.ingramcontent.com/pod-product-compliance
Lightning Source LLC
Chambersburg PA
CBHW021540260326
41914CB00001B/90